HEART
FAILURE

HEART FAILURE

FAILURE

A CRITICAL INQUIRY INTO
AMERICAN MEDICINE
AND THE REVOLUTION
IN HEART CARE

THOMAS J. MOORE

RANDOM HOUSE   NEW YORK

Library of Congress Cataloging-in-Publication Data

Moore, Thomas J.
    Heart failure: a critical inquiry into American medicine and the
    revolution in heart care / by Thomas J. Moore.
        p.   cm.
    Bibliography: p.
    ISBN 0-394-56958-X
    1. Cardiology—United States.   2. Coronary care units—United
States.   3. Medical care—United States.   I. Title.
RA645.C34M67 1989
362.1'9612'00973—dc20   88-43222

Manufactured in the United States of America
2 3 4 5 6 7 8 9
First Edition

For Barbara

ACKNOWLEDGMENTS

Only when a book is finally ready for the reader does it become apparent how much its creation depended on the generous assistance of others.

My biggest debt is to more than 300 cardiologists, heart surgeons, hospital administrators, and other professionals in the health care industry who generously shared their time, thoughts, experiences, hospitals, and operating rooms.

The main ideas in this book were tested and refined in the stimulating environment of George Washington University where I was a visiting fellow at the Graduate Institute for Policy Education and Research. I owe special thanks to Arvil V. Adams, the institute director, and Henry Solomon, dean of the Graduate School.

A group of physicians and other experts contributed greatly by reviewing portions of the manuscript for medical, factual, and logical error. They include Richard S. Snell, professor of anatomy, George Washington University; Jerold H. Theis, Department of Medical Microbiology, University of California, Davis; Joseph Lindsay, Jr., Washington Hospital Center, Washington, D.C.; Eliot Corday, Cedars-Sinai Medical Center, Los Angeles; Eugene H. Blackstone, University of Alabama at Birmingham; Robert Reis, Cedars Hospital, Miami; Craig DeAtley, EMS degree program, George Washington

University; and Henry Krakauer, Health Care Financing Administration, Baltimore. I owe a special debt to Richard W. Riegleman of George Washington University for reviewing the entire manuscript from a physician's perspective. Although it is unlikely that the reviewers will agree with everything in this book, their many comments and corrections were deeply appreciated.

The idea for this book originated in a series of articles on bypass surgery written for Knight-Ridder newspapers. I am particularly indebted to my coauthor for that series, Michael York, for his excellent reporting and for sharing many of his interview tapes. The series could not have been completed without the support of Robert S. Boyd, then the Washington Bureau Chief, and Clark Hoyt, his successor.

One way a writer can stay in touch with readers is to try out material on them frequently. I owe special thanks to these individuals for taking time to read and react to many chapters: David Bushong, Milton Carrow, Edward Krapels, and Richard Burris. Washington author David Wise contributed many valuable thoughts about the craft of book writing.

Two people at George Washington University provided invaluable practical assistance. George Paul of the Himmelfarb Health Sciences Library helped locate more than 3,000 scientific publications appearing in more than sixty medical journals, and published over fifty years' time. Further, I owe special thanks to Marcia Krueger of the Graduate Institute for her patience and assistance in preparing the manuscript.

Finally, this book would not have been possible without the advice and encouragement of one of Washington's finest investigative reporters, Seymour M. Hersh, and my editor at Random House, Robert D. Loomis.

CONTENTS

THE
HEART
AS A
FOCAL
POINT

1

TWO PATIENTS, TWO OUTCOMES

Jay H. Plotkin had just finished jogging in southwest Houston one Saturday morning when his heart abruptly stopped pumping blood. A motorist headed for the manicurist saw the fifty-four-year-old Plotkin crumple to the ground. She jumped out of the car and hollered for the neighbors to call an ambulance. Within seconds she was kneeling by Plotkin, pressing hard on his chest fifteen times, breathing into his mouth twice, then beginning the routine again.

Six minutes later paramedic Bob Schlieter had taken over the job of trying to bring Plotkin back to life. He held two paddles against Plotkin's bare chest and told everyone to stand back. Schlieter was going to use the paddles, connected to an electronic device called a defibrillator, to try to shock the heart back into operation. Plotkin's body jumped from the jolt of electricity. Still no heartbeat. Schlieter tried a second shock, and at last Plotkin's heart began to beat with disorganized and irregular contractions, but a viable pump once again. By the time Plotkin was admitted to the hospital his condition had already been stabilized.

In a coronary artery about the diameter of a pencil was a major lesion—an irregular growth of fiber and tissue somewhat like a wart. The lesion was partially obstructing the flow of blood to the most important part of the heart muscle, the left ventricle. Smaller lesions were also found elsewhere. Such blockages are frequently treated with coronary bypass surgery. Using segments of blood vessel harvested from the leg and chest, heart surgeons created a new circulatory system for Plotkin's heart. Less than one year after open-heart surgery Plotkin was jogging again.

In fifty-two active years, Susan Williamson (not her real name) never had a heart problem. The first hint of trouble came during a visit to the health club of a luxury resort. As a free service to guests the health club offered an exercise stress test, which is an electrocardiogram taken while the patient is on a treadmill. While simple and inexpensive, the stress test is not particularly accurate; in more than one out of seven cases it will indicate heart disease in perfectly healthy patients. And among women and others not at high risk it is even less reliable. Williamson tested positive. Her physician back home decided that to be on the safe side he would refer her to a cardiologist for a closer look.

Soon she was lying on a table in the cardiac catheterization laboratory of a Washington, D.C., hospital. Through an incision in her thigh, a long hollow tube was inserted into her femoral artery and threaded all the way to the heart. Special dyes were squirted through the tube to illuminate various parts of the heart while X-ray cameras recorded the results. The procedure is expensive (about $4,000) and somewhat risky, with approximately one patient in one hundred experiencing a stroke, heart attack, or other serious complication. However, it provides very exact information about the heart. Lesions had indeed formed in the network of small arteries that nourished her heart muscle with blood, but they were not as severe as Plotkin's.

At this fateful point some experts might have recommended doing nothing; she had no symptoms and might live for decades without experiencing a heart attack. Others would have proposed bypass surgery. In Williamson's case the cardiologist decided to perform balloon angioplasty, which is simpler and less drastic than open-heart surgery. A catheter was inserted in the femoral artery and gently advanced to the site of the obstruction. Then a tiny balloon was inflated to widen the narrowed place. One hazard of angioplasty is that it can accidentally block the tiny artery instead of opening it. The result is an immediate heart attack, and this was what happened to Susan Williamson. She was rushed to the operating room for emergency surgery.

A failed angioplasty is a fairly common event but often a difficult case for cardiac surgeons. When things do go badly in surgery sometimes the heart muscle becomes so inflamed and swollen that it is impossible to wire the chest closed again. And this happened to Susan Williamson. That left her heart thumping away weakly in the open chest cavity while the hospital staff waited for one thing only—for it to stop beating forever. And for Susan Williamson's now fatally damaged heart it was not a long wait.

These two cases illustrate why the human heart makes an excellent focal point to examine great achievements, and puzzle over the stark failings of modern medicine. Malfunction of the heart is the primary threat to human life in the United States today. It accounts for 36 percent of all deaths annually, dwarfing all the other major causes. Cancer, at 22 percent of deaths, is the only comparable peril. The two medical specialties of the heart, cardiology and heart surgery, are areas of such scientific vitality and clinical innovation that the most important interventions are new, either developed or perfected since 1970. The benefits of many of these new treatments have been widely heralded; the limitations and hazards have frequently been ignored. Repairing the human heart also ranks among the nation's most costly enterprises. Coronary bypass surgery, for example, has become one of the most commonly performed major operations at about the same total dollar cost as the government's entire space program. Finally, shortcomings in the practice of medicine, specially the lack of effective quality assurance, are particularly serious in coronary care because even small failings cost lives. There are moments when heart patients are some of the most fragile human beings on earth. Even the tiniest mistake can kill them.

For most of the people, most of the time, the heart is a remarkably durable fluid pump and can operate after almost 40 percent of the muscle mass has been destroyed. Outright mechanical failure of the main working parts, the four valves and chambers, is rare. However, other components of the heart are much more vulnerable. The control system that transmits the command to contract is susceptible to electrical disturbances that cause the pump to shut down abruptly, an event called sudden cardiac death; tiny arteries can become obstructed by lesions that form slowly and blood clots that appear suddenly and without warning. These vulnerabilities can produce chest pains, a heart attack or sudden death, and in medical terms are described as coronary heart disease.

Coronary heart disease was also the subject foremost in the minds of eighty-three of the nation's leading medical authorities as they gathered for a summit meeting at the National Institutes of Health in Bethesda, Maryland. The sponsor was a division of NIH called the National Heart, Lung, and Blood Institute,* and its director at the time, Robert I. Levy, was there to explain the problem that warranted this special scientific session. The year was 1978.

A striking, astounding change in deaths from coronary heart disease had occurred, Levy said. After decades of moving steadily upwards, the death rate from coronary heart disease had begun a rapid decline. In nine years the age-adjusted death rate had declined by 20 percent. That translated into 191,000 fewer deaths in a single year. In terms of human life, the magnitude of the gain was without precedent since the discovery of penicillin and other antibiotics. It was the equivalent of eliminating all the annual deaths from lung cancer, the most common malignancy.

While medical authorities have seldom been hesitant in claiming credit for improvements in the nation's health, the participants found it impossible to identify innovations in treatment to account for these enormous gains. An explosion in coronary bypass surgery had occurred beginning in 1970. But at the date of the meeting only 250,000 such operations had been performed. Even in the improbable event that each one had saved a life, bypass surgery couldn't account for a fraction of the change. A slightly older innovation was coronary intensive care units, which in some hospitals had seemed to bring dramatic reductions in heart attack deaths. But since most such deaths occur quickly, and

*For simplicity the National Heart, Lung, and Blood Institute will be hereafter identified as the heart institute.

before hospital admission, the special units could only have saved a small fraction of the total.

If better medical treatment could not account for the gain, perhaps sweeping changes in the nation's lifestyles were responsible. But the experts who studied specific risk factors, such as diet, smoking, and high blood pressure, simply could not identify big enough shifts to account for the decline. It seemed clear the population had healthier hearts, but specific reasons for this welcome change remained a mystery.

By 1986 the overall decline in heart disease deaths was more dramatic yet, and reasons were no clearer. At another conference of experts, Thomas Thom, an epidemiologist and a world authority on the incidence of heart disease, reported that the death rate had now declined 42 percent from the peak year, pinpointed as 1963. However dramatic that might be, Thom said, "The state of our knowledge about why the decline is occurring is improving very undramatically."

The conferences illustrate the curious combination of achievement and failure that will be found repeatedly in American medicine's response to the principal peril to life. The participants could rightfully take pride in the vigor of their assault, including a daring new surgical treatment, specialized hospital units, and a massive public health campaign against risk factors. Nevertheless, it had taken eight years before the nation's principal authorities had detected a monumental change in the health status of America. And twenty-three years after that trend began, the reasons still could not be explained. What if the trend had run in the opposite direction and it had taken eight years to detect a rapid increase in deaths? How confident can we be in the management of a vast and expensive effort when the costs, gains, and losses are not being systematically measured? The reasons for and consequences of this important shortcoming will form a major focus of this book.

The reasons for both successes and failures in medicine today are often reflected most clearly not in the outcome of individual cases, but in key decisions that affect the health and treatment of millions of Americans. The logic behind one such pivotal decision can be seen in an important medical experiment.

A carefully screened group of 143 men agreed to join a five-year government study. While the subjects had no symptoms of ill health, the medical investigators believed the volunteers were at increased risk of death or serious injury, and sought scientific evidence they could reduce that risk. As each subject was entered into the experiment, a researcher selected at random a sealed envelope. The contents would determine whether the participant would take two drugs every day or get identical-looking placebos.

Less than half way through the intended treatment period the Veterans Administration investigators abruptly terminated the experiment. They already had recorded an appalling number of adverse events, twenty-nine in all. Four men had died, including three whose aorta, the largest blood vessel in the body, had suddenly ruptured. Two had experienced heart attacks and five more suffered strokes. In others, tiny blood vessels in the eye were beginning to hemorrhage.

All the adverse events except two had occurred in the placebo group. This was such compelling evidence for the effect of treatment that it was unethical to withhold the benefits of the medication from the controls.

The year was 1967, and all the participants had a condition that is usually without symptoms but not without great hazard to life: They had severely elevated blood pressure. This experiment provided an important part of the scientific foundation for a vast public campaign to identify millions of Americans with high blood pressure and treat them in hopes of preventing future heart attacks, strokes, and other injury. More than two decades later the treatment of hypertension would account for more office visits to doctors than any condition except the common cold. At a cost of four billion dollars annually more than nineteen million people take blood pressure medication daily.

Almost no program of preventive medicine is without risks as well as benefits, and the treatment of hypertension was no exception. Evidence has since accumulated that about one quarter of those on hypertension drugs experienced adverse effects, including impotence, fatigue, lethargy, and elevated blood cholesterol.* As a result, many patients wouldn't take their medication. In response, the government spent millions studying psychological techniques to induce the reluctant to take the medicine. And while the benefits were incontestable

---

*Adverse effects also vary widely among the various kinds of hypertension drugs.

for severely high blood pressure, a lively scientific debate continues about the wisdom of the current policy of treating the millions with much more moderate elevations.

The hypertension program illustrates many of the provocative questions that arise in the prevention of coronary heart disease. Almost any adult can explain the process by which income taxes are raised, a certain behavior declared illegal, or tax dollars expended. But what is the nature of the process that determines that millions of Americans without symptoms are at risk and require expensive medical treatment? What kind of scientific evidence is required? How are adverse effects monitored and the benefits measured? Is the new assault on cholesterol built on as solid a scientific foundation as the campaign against hypertension?

If prevention fails, the alternative is more drastic medical or surgical treatment of patients whose initial problem may range from mild warning symptoms to an immediately life-threatening crisis. Treatment raises a separate set of questions which are illustrated in an operation that involves many of the same issues as bypass surgery.

A fifty-three-year-old school bus driver lay unconscious on the operating room table before surgeon Michael DeBakey, who was about to begin a procedure he had never performed before. The same process that causes lesions to form in the coronary arteries also creates irregular growths in other blood vessels. And DeBakey's target was a blockage in the left common carotid, an artery in the neck that is almost as critical as those that supply the heart. Compared to the tiny coronary arteries, the carotid is large and easily accessible. But on this day in August 1953 few surgeons had yet dared to try this procedure on such an essential blood vessel. DeBakey had informed his patient of the pioneering character of the operation, but in the confident manner of surgeons, he described the risk as "slight."

Soon DeBakey had exposed a segment of the left carotid just at the point where it first divides into two major branches. He closed a clamp over the artery to stop the flow of blood. After a quick, sure incision, the interior of the blood vessel lay open to view. Right at the junction, masses of firm yellowish-brown material had nearly halted the flow of blood. And a fresh blood clot had formed at the already narrowed site, totally obstructing one of the branches. These were doubtless the reasons why the patient had experienced weakness and numbness in one arm and occasional difficulty speaking. DeBakey quickly removed the fresh blood clot and separated the older mass of fiber, plaque, and tissue from the blood vessel wall. Then he stitched the artery closed again with fine silk thread. In one of the earliest of DeBakey's pioneering contributions to surgery he had just performed one of the earliest successful attempts at an operation that would be called a carotid endarterectomy (EN-darter-ectomy). It also paved the way towards the enormously more demanding operations on arteries of the human heart.

As testimony that even the towering figures in heart surgery are not infallible DeBakey was proved dead wrong on one important point. When the operation spread into clinical use the risks proved to be anything but "slight." For example, a 1984 study of all such procedures performed in Cincinnati in one year showed that one out of ten patients either died or suffered a stroke, the event the operation was intended to prevent. Equally disturbing was a 1988 Rand Corporation examination of the operation as performed by 236 surgeons on 1,390 Medicare patients in three separate geographic areas. Following the operation, a total of 11.6 percent of the patients were dead, suffered permanent brain damage from a stroke, or experienced a heart attack.

The risks proved so great that a policy committee of the American Neurological Association questioned the value of the operation since it may have caused more deaths and strokes than it prevented. "We conclude that the procedure may be of value if the surgical complication rate is very low, but that the net effect in the United States as a whole may be unfavorable." Whatever the committee's opinion, the carotid endarterectomy is one of the most frequently performed major operations today. More than 100,000 such procedures are performed each year.

Thus the carotid endarterectomy illustrates some of the questions that must be asked about the equally demanding treatments for the human heart. What are the major therapies and how well do they work? What kind of system controls the invention, testing, and introduction of new surgical procedures and other potentially hazardous treatments? How often are dangerous operations performed on persons likely to receive little or no benefit, or for whom the benefits are uncertain?

• • •

In April 1985 a little-noticed decision by the federal government provided outsiders with the first peek into one of the most closely held secrets of hospitals. The government declared that hospital-specific information about the costs and treatment of Medicare patients was available to the public providing it did not invade the privacy of the doctor/patient relationship. Analysts in government, the universities, and the news media quickly realized that it was now possible to compare hospitals in new and provocative ways. One was to compare deaths from open-heart surgery. Within a hospital such mortality data was so tightly held it was normally known only to the cardiac surgeons and a handful of others. And outside the hospital such figures were virtually unobtainable, except from a few famous medical centers which prided themselves on routine publication of their surgical results. The first government figures, while limited to the 40 percent of bypass operations paid for by Medicare, painted a startling picture.

In New York City, Lenox Hill Hospital serves the fashionable clientele of the upper East Side, and offered open-heart surgery under its chief cardiac surgeon, Eugene Wallsh. In 1984 coronary bypass operations were performed on fifty-nine Medicare patients at a mortality rate of 15.2 percent, according to the federal data. In all, nine Medicare patients died after surgery.

On the opposite coast the Eisenhower Medical Center provides hospital care to the residents of affluent Rancho Mirage, a next-door neighbor to the Palm Springs resort community. Open-heart surgery at Eisenhower was performed by Jack J. Sternlieb, who in 1984 performed bypass surgery on 161 Medicare patients. Just one patient died, for a mortality rate of less than 1 percent. Thus it appeared that a Medicare patient was fifteen times more likely to die after bypass surgery at Lenox Hill than at Eisenhower Medical Center.

As far as could be determined the patients at the two hospitals were fairly similar. For example, advancing age significantly increases the risk of bypass surgery. Sternlieb's bypass patients in California were typically older than those at Lenox Hill even though fewer died. Interviews with both surgeons revealed no unusual differences in patients that would immediately explain the large difference in mortality. However, Wallsh said, "There are patients who are operated on here who probably wouldn't be operated on in another hospital because they were too sick." But Sternlieb's assessment of his own surgical practice was little different. "We take all comers who can benefit from the operation. We don't exclude patients for high risk because of old age or previous damage to their heart."

The magnitude of such differences was not lost on the medical authorities at Lenox Hill, which retained the famed heart surgeon John W. Kirklin to evaluate the hospital's heart surgery program. The results of that examination have not been disclosed. But Wallsh was replaced as chief cardiac surgeon. In its first year of operation the new surgical team reported a mortality rate of 1.8 percent among Medicare patients.

Sometimes these dramatic contrasts extend to entire cities. In Fort Wayne, Indiana, and Las Vegas, Nevada, a similar volume of bypass surgery was performed on Medicare patients in 1984. In Fort Wayne just two patient deaths occurred in 196 operations. In Las Vegas there were twenty-eight deaths among 194 bypass patients. Because such comparisons had never been possible before the federal government began to release the data, the surgeons in Las Vegas seemed completely unaware of the city's high death rate for bypass surgery. "Look, we can't all be jerks," said one of the city's heart surgeons.

So why do the results of demanding treatments such as heart surgery vary so widely among hospitals? Are they because of the kind of the patients who went to surgery? Can the real explanation be found in the skills of the surgeons or the quality of the hospital? What happens inside a hospital when the mortality rate begins to climb? How effective is the system to detect and correct mistakes in medicine when dealing with the complex and demanding task of heart surgery?

This book cannot hope to meet the special requirements of those who need health advice about their heart. Individual circumstances vary too widely to place this subject within the legitimate scope of this analysis. However, it may nevertheless provide a basis for informed questions about the coronary care that is proposed, and a realistic understanding of the people and institutions that will provide that care.

When this examination of medicine and the human heart began in 1986 I experienced a powerful emotion that I had not felt for nearly twenty years. The last time was as a young Army officer in Vietnam.

It was like arriving on a strange new planet where an entirely new set of rules applied and all previous experience in a gentler world became of dubious relevance. Because life itself is at stake, the world of a failing human heart transforms one's entire perspective in a similar way. Even though they may live next door, the men and women who must deal with these problems every day inhabit a starkly different world. This book is an effort to portray it.

2
HEARTS THEN
AND NOW

It goes to work long before you are born. When it stops the rest of your life can be measured in minutes. As the cells of a human embryo divide and begin to specialize after conception, the first rudimentary organ to take shape is the heart. The earliest contractions begin the third week after conception. Interruption of the heart's regular output for more than a few seconds causes loss of consciousness; death occurs within six to twelve minutes. Not only is uninterrupted operation essential, the heart is loaded with complicated moving parts, and tucked safely away in one of the most inaccessible locations in the body. When something does go wrong, repair is not a simple job.

The human heart consists of two pumps joined together on a fibrous skeleton. In the language of engineering it is a two-cylinder reciprocating fluid pump mounted on a flexible chassis. The main pump drives blood around the body; another supplies the lungs. The blood pressure levels in the rest of the body would quickly rupture the 400 million tiny sacs in the lungs where carbon dioxide and oxygen are exchanged. These delicate sacs have such an enormous surface area that if flattened out they would cover an area the size of a tennis court. Consequently, a separate pump operating at one sixth the pressure in the rest of the body drives blood through the lungs. In an adult male the entire heart assembly is slightly larger than the clenched fist and weighs about two thirds of a pound. Daily it puts forth a prodigious effort, performing the equivalent labor of hoisting the entire body to the top of a forty-story building. In normal operation the two pumps' combined output totals about a gallon a minute, and rises to five gallons a minute during strenuous exercise.

The structure of the two pumps is similar: a small chamber, or atrium, to collect the return flow of blood, and a larger pumping chamber called a ventricle. Despite a gallon-a-minute throughput, the chambers that collect the return flow are surprisingly small, each with a capacity of about two ounces. The small size suffices because the blood flows directly into the larger ventricle during most of the pumping cycle.

The right ventricle, the low pressure pump supplying the lungs, has thin walls but holds the same volume as the real workhorse of the heart, the left ventricle. Nearly three quarters of the muscle mass is devoted to this thick-walled chamber. Most of the clinical measures of heart function concern the performance of the left ventricle. Heart failure in medical terminology means inability to pump enough blood to the rest of the body. Most often that involves irreversible damage to the left ventricle.

While the heart is a straightforward, two-cylinder fluid pump, nearly 2,000 years of recorded medical history passed before physicians correctly understood its function. A physician's son named Aristotle was among the earliest influential thinkers to set forth his ideas in detail. His concepts of government and politics remain respectable today, but he was hopelessly confused about the heart. In Aristotle's view the heart was the seat of life and the origin of all emotions and where the voice originated. The brain, in his scheme, served mainly to cool the blood. Like other early Greeks he believed the arteries contained air, a particularly potent vapor called life pneuma, rather than blood.

Aristotle and other early Greeks' misconceptions remain embedded in the language to this day. A broken heart is more likely to refer to an emotional state than to difficulties pumping blood. Aristotle, ordinarily a most astute observer of life and nature, worked under a significant disadvantage because it was a sacrilege to dissect the human body.

A few decades later another famed Greek physician, Erasistratus, labored under no such restrictions in his studies at Alexandria, the ancient world's most important center of learning. He not only dissected cadavers but cut apart condemned criminals while still alive. He left detailed descriptions of the ventricles of the heart and valves. Aristotle and other early Greeks believed the arteries contained air because they were in fact empty of blood when they dissected dead animals. The arteries are elastic and contract at death, while the non-elastic veins remain open and thus retain blood. Erasistratus, however, found plenty of blood in the arteries when he cut into them during his ghoulish experiments. But what was blood doing in the vessels supposed to contain life pneuma? He explained this by postulating the existence of invisible connections that allowed the blood to rush from the veins into the arteries only when the arteries were punctured—as for example during his experiments. Under normal circumstances the arteries still contained air as Aristotle had decreed. Erasistratus was neither the first nor last medical thinker to invent non-existent anatomical features to reconcile what he saw with the authoritative view.

Erasistratus' ideas guided the medical world for centuries until extensively revised by the medical giant of Roman times, Claudius Galenus, or Galen. He was personal physician to Emperor Marcus Aurelius and successors, and a towering medical authority in his own day. He dissected animals at well-attended public lectures, heaped scorn on the ignorance of his competitors and colleagues, and left behind a major body of medical literature, including fifteen books of anatomy. His descriptions were crisp, clear, complete, and in the case of the heart, erroneous. By tying ligatures around arteries and then determining their contents, he correctly concluded they contained blood. He observed that both the right and left ventricles contracted to expel blood. But Galen misunderstood the function of the lungs. He believed that air and blood were combined in the left ventricle, and the air entered the ventricle through the pulmonary veins. That scheme, however, leaves a major problem. If it is air that enters the heart through the pulmonary veins connected to the lungs, then how does the blood get there? In Galen's scheme blood moved from the right ventricle directly to the left ventricle through invisible pores in the solid mass of muscle and fiber that divides the two main pumping chambers.

For nearly a thousand years Galen's books were the unquestioned authority on the practice of medicine and the functions of the human body, including the heart. Even in the Renaissance when dissections were again allowed for medical school training Galen's texts still held uncontested sway. Period paintings show anatomy classes with the professor on a raised platform with a text of Galen while below a barber displays the appropriate organ. Nobody seemed to notice that the human sternum and liver looked quite different from what was shown in Galen's text, which was based on animal rather than human anatomy. The apparent failure of anyone to note the difference stands as another testament to the human animal's frequent tendency to see only what it wants to see, and to the enduring influence of the authoritative text in medicine. By the 1530s Andreas Vesalius, an anatomist so passionate that he would analyze the chicken bones on his dinner plate, began correcting the worst of Galen's errors. However, Vesalius couldn't find any trace of the pores through which blood flowed from the left to the right ventricle. While Vesalius was willing to attack other Galen errors, he missed the idea of blood circulation through the lungs:

"We are obliged to wonder at the unseen work of the Creator through which blood travels by unseen roads from the right to left ventricle."

However, some old-guard medical school professors clung tightly to the historical authority of Galen. One even insisted that Galen was perfectly accurate; it was the body that had changed under the influence of dissolute Renaissance living.

The first physician credited with getting the basic scheme correct was a rebellious and freethinking Spaniard named Michael Servetus. At the height of the Inquisition and the extraordinary religious tensions of the reformation Servetus succeeded in antagonizing both Catholics and John Calvin's early Protestants with a heretical analysis of the Holy Trinity. The work got him burned at the stake. But in the middle of his 1546 religious tract was a digression that correctly described the functions of the chambers of the heart. He saw that the right ventricle pumped blood into the lungs, that the blood returned in the pulmonary veins to the left atrium. So there for the first time in recorded history was the basic idea of how the heart worked, inserted as Chapter Five in the heretical tract "Errors of the Holy Trinity."

While Servetus had the right idea, his thinking was not widely circulated. It was an additional seventy years before William Harvey formally proposed the circulation of blood, probably in a 1615 lecture to the College of Physicians in London. Harvey's detailed and authoritative exposition left two important loose ends. He thought that the function of the lungs was to cool the blood rather than oxygenate it. And there was no clear account of how the blood got from the arteries and back into the veins.

It is easy to understand how early physicians had trouble with these two ideas until Anton van Leeuwenhoek's invention of the microscope allowed scientists to see features invisible to the naked eye. With one of the early microscopes Italian anatomist Marcello Malpighi was able to observe the blood being oxygenated in the tiny capillaries in the lungs of a frog. And with a microscope the capillaries elsewhere in the body could be identified and their function at last deduced. Thus Hippocrates recorded the symptoms of a heart attack ("Sharp pains irradiating soon towards the clavicle and back are fatal.") But another 2,000 years passed before scientists understood how the heart worked.

The familiar "lubb-dup" of the heartbeat is not the muscle contracting. The sounds are created by the valves snapping shut. In the right heart the three leaflets of the tricuspid valve separate the atrium where the return flow of blood collects from the ventricle, the pumping chamber. When the heart begins to contract, the increasing pressure snaps the valve shut. As the heart muscle relaxes, the three leaflets fall open, and blood floods from the atrium into the ventricle. It is a large valve for a large opening—wide enough to admit the tips of four fingers. Each of the leaflets of the valve is anchored by thin tendons that look like parachute cords connected to pillars of muscle rising from inside the ventricle. The cords don't control the valve, they just secure the leaflets in the closed position while the heart is contracting. In the left ventricle the mitral valve is similarly constructed, except it is half as big in area and has only two leaflets.

At the exits of both ventricles are valves that serve the same basic purpose as the valve on a bicycle tire while being inflated. The valve maintains the pressure in the tire between strokes of the pump, but passes the air from the pump into the tire while the pump pressure is higher. The pulmonary valve performs the same job for the artery leading to the lungs, and the aortic valve maintains blood pressure for the rest of the body. Thus the first of the heart sounds is the tricuspid and mitral valves snapping shut as the contraction begins. The short second sound is the pulmonary and aortic valves snapping shut after pumping blood to the lungs and body.

The valves, which open and close thirty-eight million times a year, rank among the most continuously stressed mechanical moving parts in the body. But their overall record of durability is exceptional. Rheumatic fever, once among the most dangerous diseases of childhood, often left in its wake a "heart murmur," which usually signalled permanent damage to the mitral valve. The disease left portions of the leaflets scarred and fused together, and sometimes damaged the delicate tendons that secure the leaflets. With the near disappearance of rheumatic fever, valve malfunctions now mostly affect the very young and the elderly. In infants the valves may be malformed at birth; among the elderly, deposits of calcium can narrow the valve opening, or prevent a tight closure. Defective valves can be replaced with artificial models fashioned from the hearts of pigs, or by metal and plastic devices. Valve replacement is a difficult and relatively risky operation, but is performed thousands of times every year.

However unique the size and capability of man's brain, humans were nevertheless issued the standard model mammalian heart. Except for size, only an expert in comparative heart anatomy could tell the difference between the one-ounce rat heart, the twelve-ounce human version and the nine-pound horse model. All have four-chambered hearts with the same arrangement of valves. Generally blood pressure is about the same in mammals of all sizes because of a common purpose: It must be high enough to force the blood through capillary blood vessels of microscopic size. As a result, in a smaller animal the reduced-size heart must beat a lot faster to achieve the necessary blood pressure. Therefore a rat heart beats at about 328 beats a minute, a human heart at 70, and an elephant just 35. The differences at the extremes are even more dramatic: The pinhead-sized heart of the hummingbird has been clocked at 1,000 beats a minute. The giant model is found in the sixty-five-foot long adult male sperm whale, whose heart is about the size of a washing machine. It beats only twelve times a minute on the surface, and perhaps one beat a minute when submerged.

Creatures farther down the evolutionary tree have related but simpler hearts. Fish, for example, have a one-cylinder heart rather than the mammals' two-cylinder model. They do, however, have an atrium, a valve, and a ventricle for pumping. To prevent damage to the delicate gills some fish have a flexible, balloon-like structure connected to the heart that inflates with each heartbeat, thereby smoothing the blood flow. In human beings the elastic arteries perform a similar function.

Amphibians, with their primitive lungs, may have the strangest of all arrangements. Like humans they have two atria, one to collect deoxygenated blood from the body, and another to collect blood from the lungs. But amphibians have just one ventricle to pump the blood. Through an ingenious arrangement and careful timing, the blood awaiting oxygenation ends up in the ventricle, on top of the already oxygenated blood. When the single ventricle contracts, the first blood expelled flows down the pulmonary arteries to the rudimentary lungs. The rest of the ventricle's contents, the oxygenated blood, is pumped on to the rest of the body.

The rhythmic tracings from the twelve leads of the electrocardiogram hint at the rich and complex electrical activity of the heart. Tiny electrical currents in the individual muscle cells of the heart enable them to contract automatically like microscopic robots. Furthermore, the muscle fibers are bundled tightly together so that when one cell is electrically excited it also stimulates its neighbors to contract. However, getting the complicated, four-chambered pump to operate properly requires more elaborate overall coordination and timing. The cells must not only contract regularly, but in a particular sequence and at varying speeds. To accomplish this the heart cells must march to the beat of a common drummer, a tiny patch of cells normally located on the front wall of the right atrium. Called the pacemaker of the heart, this patch of tissue contracts at the normal resting heart rate of approximately seventy beats per minute. Each contraction of these cells sends an electrical impulse that ripples across the common muscle fibers of the right and left atria. As the impulse moves across the muscles, each atrium contracts, emptying the last of its contents into the ventricles.

A fraction of a second later the signal arrives at another specialized patch of cells, the A-V node, responsible for timing and forwarding the impulse to trigger the contraction of the ventricles. To get a powerful contraction, the muscle fibers of the ventricles must contract nearly simultaneously, rather than allowing the impulse to ripple more gradually from cell to cell. Another network of specialized cells, operating almost like electrical wiring, rapidly transmits the command to contract to the muscle cells throughout the left and right ventricles. The ventricles contract almost in unison, and blood is pumped to the lungs and the rest of the body. When the electrical impulses are mapped out on an electrocardiogram, the line tracing shows a gradual hump as the left and right atrium contract, followed by an enormous spike as the impulse is rapidly transmitted to the muscle fibers that spiral around the ventricles.

At a resting heart rate of seventy beats per minute this system will work without any outside involvement or control. In fact, when removed entirely from the body the heart continues to beat for several minutes; with rudimentary nutrients it will beat for hours outside the body. However, the heart is a pump capable of large variations in output. These variations are mainly controlled by signals from the brain that travel down two separate nerve pathways to release hormones that reduce or enormously increase the heart's output. One hormone not only can triple the pulse rate, but also can double the strength of the contractions. At the other extreme, the hormone that slows the heart rate is so powerful that it can suppress the heartbeat entirely for a few seconds. Finally, the heart has another characteristic that adds to its flexibility as a pump. As the heart is filled with greater quantities of blood, the muscle fibers are stretched. And when so stretched they contract with additional force. This gives the heart the capability of pumping widely varying quantities of blood in a single contraction.

Electrical activity was not only the last major heart function to be understood, but a complete explanation of one critical problem still eludes medical science: Why is the electrical system of the heart so easily disrupted? If the carefully timed rhythmic pulses are disturbed, the muscle fibers can begin to contract chaotically and spontaneously, a condition called fibrillation. The flow of blood halts, and unconsciousness and death rapidly follow. It ranks among the few common medical conditions that, without intervention, are invariably fatal, claiming 300,000 lives each year. However, the condition that ranks as one of the nation's major causes of death is also readily reversed. A brief electric shock instantly resets the electrical system of the heart and restores the heartbeat. The problem is time. Irreversible brain damage occurs so rapidly that the correct shock must be administered within a few minutes of the event.

The heart muscle ought to be the last of all places in the human body to have trouble getting an adequate supply of blood, but that is the central problem of the pump. It's simply not enough to have the four heart chambers usually filled with blood. Oxygen and nutrients must be delivered directly to the individual cells through a network of tiny arteries that divide into smaller and smaller branches until they are barely bigger in diameter than a single red blood cell.

Blood reaches the heart muscle itself through two small arteries. The left main coronary artery is a blood vessel about the size of the little finger. It soon divides into two important branches that supply practically all of the blood needed to sustain the main power pump, the left ventricle. The opposite side of the heart is supplied by the smaller right coronary artery. The overall arrangement, however, is neither tidy nor uniform from person to person. In some individuals the right coronary artery supplies almost half the heart's blood; in most others the left main coronary artery plays the dominant role. After delivering oxygen and nutrients through microscopic-sized capillaries, the return flow of blood is collected in a roughly parallel set of veins and dumped directly back into the right atrium of the heart.

The heart's network of tiny arteries is critical. It delivers oxygen and fuel to power the pump, drains off many waste products, and provides the raw materials needed for cell maintenance. Compared to other organs and muscles, the coronary arteries must deliver an unusually large volume of blood under high pressure. Unfortunately, they are also vulnerable to developing obstructions.

Blockages in the coronary arteries can be large or small, partial or complete, form quickly or over many years. Frequently irregular growths called lesions slowly form near major branch points, possibly a response to injury to the vessel wall from the high pressure flow. Three severe medical problems are linked to these lesions. Over years the lesions may grow large enough to prevent the heart from obtaining an extra supply of blood when needed, for example during exercise. This causes temporary oxygen starvation, and sometimes chest pain, but no permanent damage. A more serious problem can begin when a lesion ruptures or breaks open. A blood clot suddenly forms at the site and it can obstruct the artery, halting the flow entirely. When an area of heart tissue is suddenly deprived entirely of blood the muscle cells die in about an hour's time. This is the classic heart attack, or in medical terms, an acute myocardial infarction, meaning sudden death of heart muscle tissue. The dead cells are ultimately replaced by non-functional scar tissue, but the damage to the heart is irreversible. Finally, it is perhaps temporary oxygen starvation caused by a lesion that triggers most episodes of the deadly electrical disorder of ventricular fibrillation, but the exact mechanism remains unknown.

Not only are the coronary arteries the most vulnerable feature of the heart, they are a major challenge to repair. The valves and chambers are large and visible features. But the network of tiny arteries is a technical nightmare. It is difficult to find the blockages and even harder to eliminate them. Once removed the obstructions tend to recur. The process by which these irregular growths form is imperfectly understood, and the techniques for removing them are crude and only partially effective at best. Since life literally depends on these arteries they form the principal focus for medical maintenance of the heart. And the ideal approach would be to prevent them from becoming obstructed in the first place.

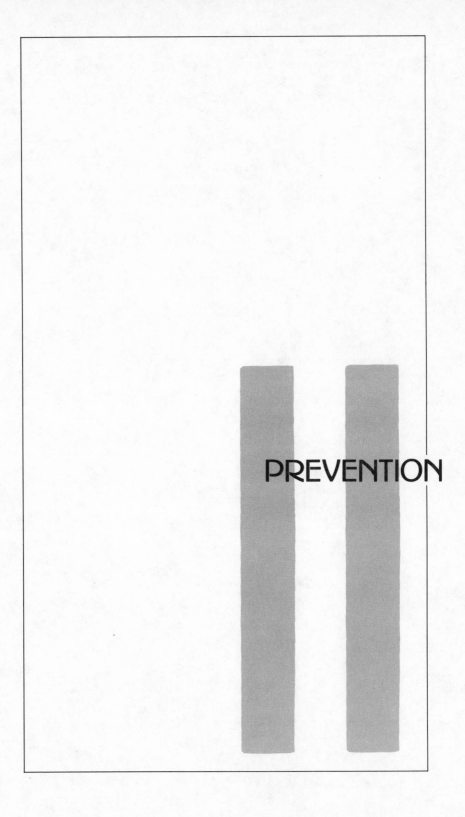

PREVENTION

3
THE CAMPAIGN BEGINS

One morning in early October 1987 the U.S. health authorities announced that 25 percent of the adult population had a dangerous condition requiring medical treatment. Since there were no symptoms it would be necessary to screen the entire population to identify those in danger. More than half would be dispatched to their physicians for additional medical tests and evaluation. Then for one out of four adults treatment would begin. The first step would be a strict diet under medical supervision. If within three months the dieting had not achieved specific results that could be verified by laboratory tests, a more severe diet would be imposed. The final step for many patients would be powerful drugs to be taken for the rest of their lives.

Considering that it was expected to become one of the most massive medical interventions in the nation's history, the formal announcement was deceptively low key. It was to be called the National Cholesterol Education Program. And while cholesterol was surely a household word, the official sponsor was less familiar: the National Heart, Lung, and Blood Institute, a major division of the federal government's National Institutes of Health. While the heart institute's main job is to coordinate and finance medical research, this departure into massive medical intervention was unusual but not unprecedented. And at first glance the program's objective sounded positively innocuous: "To reduce the prevalence of elevated blood cholesterol in the United States and thereby contribute to reducing coronary heart disease morbidity and mortality." However, despite an initially low public profile, the National Cholesterol Education Program was a medical landmark on several grounds.

It was the culmination of an extraordinary and sustained medical research effort targeted against the nation's biggest killer, coronary heart disease. One experiment took forty years and was still going. Another involved 361,622 middle-aged men. One of the most famous experiments, by two Nobel Prize winners, had penetrated to the innermost recesses of the human cell to identify a single gene with a dramatic effect on cholesterol levels. Researchers had studied rabbits, fed high-fat diets to monkeys and egg yolks to college students. It would be hard to find another medical question that had been explored with such vigor, by so many researchers, and at such great expense. Just two important experiments took twelve years, cost more than $300 million, and consumed 60 percent of the heart institute's clinical research budget.

There were also serious risks to consider. Not since the introduction of oral contraceptives might so many people be exposed to powerful new prescription drugs for decades, if not their lifetimes. One of the most elusive hazards of drugs is the toxic effects that emerge only after being administered to thousands of people for years. Some side effects are extremely serious, but rare enough that they are not discovered until after a drug is placed in wide use. Other ill-effects may occur frequently but cannot be detected except after years of exposure. Nor was dietary therapy quite as simple as it looked. So complex are the interactions among specific food compounds and so varied is the behavior and chemistry of individuals that dietary intervention had proved to be one of the most complicated of all medical treatments. History is filled with accounts of unexpected side effects or disappointing results.

Finally, the National Cholesterol Education Program represented a major change in strategy in the prevention of coronary heart disease. Previous efforts, led mainly by the American Heart Association, relied on advice and persuasion. Now the federal government was going to call on the authority of physicians to prescribe a medically supervised regimen of treatment. This was not just friendly advice from the family doctor to cut down on cholesterol. It was, in the words of the treatment guidelines, a program of "behavior modification" backed by laboratory tests to insure adherence and measure results. People might abandon drugs that made them sick—and some cholesterol-lowering drugs were famous for this effect—or refuse to eat foods they didn't like. But now they would be violating explicit doctors' orders.

Before a government program of such importance moved into high gear one would expect it to have first survived extensive scrutiny. One would suppose that such a far-reaching intervention into the lives of millions of people would have been approved by the White House and scrutinized by Congress. In fact, the heart institute launched this project on its own authority, consulting mainly with special panels of hand-picked physicians. One would suppose that before putting millions of people on a medically supervised diet it would have been tested in advance to demonstrate that it was safe and that it worked. No such tests were conducted. One would suppose that the nation's clinical laboratories could measure cholesterol accurately enough to identify those who needed treatment. In fact, laboratory performance was so poor that millions with average or low blood cholesterol would be misled into believing their levels were dangerously high. One would suppose that before launching a program that would involve billions of dollars in doctors' bills, laboratory tests and medication, the costs and benefits would have been carefully weighed. In reality, officials would not even guess at the total costs and had no plan to measure the benefits. And one would suppose that it had been conclusively demonstrated that lowering blood cholesterol would save lives. No such evidence existed. The story begins in 1953 when Army and Marine Corps doctors published a discovery that shocked the medical world.

• • •

SOON AFTER THE Korean War began the Pentagon dispatched a team of pathologists to the combat zone for the grisly mission of learning from the bodies of the dead. Their principal assignment was to examine wound ballistics, and over three years they performed autopsies on 2,000 dead soldiers. As a group, battle casualties differ greatly from the subjects a pathologist normally examines, who are mostly old and very sick. However, until their lives were abruptly terminated, these soldiers were the flower of youth. But as Major William F. Enos and Lieutenant Colonel Robert H. Holmes performed their autopsies they began to notice signs of coronary heart disease in these vigorous young men. This was surprising because practically nobody under thirty-five dies of coronary heart disease and these war dead were, on the average, twenty-two years old. So the pathologists launched a systematic study of the hearts of the battle casualties. For 300 consecutive cases they methodically dissected the single most vulnerable component of the heart, the network of tiny coronary arteries that nourish the muscle with blood.

These small arteries are considerably more sophisticated than just hollow tubes through which the heart's blood supply flows. The inside surface is a thin layer of very smooth, almost slick cells. It needs to be smooth for a specific purpose. The platelets and proteins in the blood are constantly seeking any break or irregularity, and when they encounter one lay down a deposit of fibrous material. Such a fibrous deposit on the skin is the familiar scab. The next major layer in the artery consists of smooth muscle which can expand and contract like other muscles in the body. One of the mechanisms by which the heart muscle can increase its blood supply is by dilating the coronary arteries, thus increasing the flow.

So when the military pathologists began to dissect the coronary arteries of the combat casualties they expected to find mostly slick interior surfaces surrounded by healthy smooth muscle. What they actually found was something quite different. In 35 percent of the casualties the inner surface of the arteries already showed early evidence of coronary heart disease. Instead of a smooth surface they found stringy, streaky yellow deposits of fats and fiber. These particular deposits were no immediate threat. But it meant that degeneration of the arteries was well under way on a wide scale more than twenty years before these men would normally experience heart attacks.

In another 42 percent of the casualties the coronary arteries were in even worse shape. In this group the fatty streaks had already grown into full-fledged lesions, structures that somewhat resemble a wart on the skin. The lesion is usually capped by a hard, fibrous plaque. Inside is a mass of debris that can include cholesterol compounds, dead tissue, and calcium. Some lesions are soft, like pimples; others are hard as a rock. Once these lesions get established they slowly increase in size. Fortunately for human life expectancy, they can block about 75 percent of the diameter of the artery without seriously inhibiting the blood flow. Further, some areas of the heart muscle are nourished by more than one branch of the network of arteries. So as one artery slowly becomes blocked, the tissue can sometimes get blood through another. One out of ten soldiers already had lesions severe enough to reduce or block entirely the flow of blood in at least one artery.

These men's arteries were in terrible shape. A total of 77 percent of the Korean casualties examined showed gross evidence of coronary heart disease, and in 1953 this was a shock to the medical community for several reasons. It meant that the process underlying coronary heart disease began much earlier than anyone thought. Here were fully developed lesions, some entirely obstructing arteries, in twenty-two-year-olds. Furthermore, practically everyone had at least some signs of coronary heart disease.

These lesions would remain at the center of medical interest in coronary heart disease for decades to come. Cholesterol-lowering diets would aim to slow their growth; bypass surgery would attempt to route blood around them; balloon angioplasty, to squeeze the lesions open. All this intense interest came because if, at the site of these lesions, the blood flow were suddenly halted, the affected area of the heart muscle would die. But in 1953 researchers faced a more immediate problem. Without examining the coronary arteries directly, how were physicians going to tell who was in danger? The answer to that question was just then beginning to take shape eighteen miles west of Boston in an industrial town called Framingham.

• • •

IF PHYSICIANS COULD pinpoint what was different about the people with coronary heart disease, maybe they could learn to save them. But in a free-living population, tracing the development of such an elusive but universal peril was a formidable scientific task. It would require careful and systematic surveillance of thousands of people for years on end. One might as well examine the population of an entire city, and that is exactly the task that a team of Boston University Medical School physicians undertook in Framingham, Massachusetts. It was among the heart institute's first massive projects. The researchers, led by Boston University's Thomas R. Dawber, hoped to recruit most of the adult population of Framingham and study them for the rest of their lives. The project, which continues to this day, began in 1948.

The first disappointment came not long after they set up shop in the mostly blue-collar community of 28,000, of mostly ethnic Irish and Italians. They hoped to recruit two out of every three healthy adults from age thirty to sixty-two. As the team selected the subjects, however, they were surprised to discover that more than one third of those invited to participate refused. This large group obviously did not want to undergo physical examinations, fill out detailed questionnaires about their living habits and diet, and be tested with exercise treadmills and electrocardiograms. The battery of tests would consume almost a full morning of time and would be repeated every two years. The study team held worried discussions about whether the experiment was doomed from the start because the one third who declined to participate might also share other important traits. If this made their sample unrepresentative, it might distort any conclusions they might later reach. However, the team decided to recruit additional volunteers, and were soon ready to observe what happened to 5,127 healthy men and women.

Probably in no other city in the United States were a population's health, weight, diet, exercise, and living habits measured so systematically for so many years. A substantial fraction of everything that medical science knows today about the epidemiology of coronary heart disease was learned from the residents of Framingham. But the events that unfolded over the next thirty years were heavily influenced by the strengths—and major weaknesses—of the particular kind of knowledge that emerges from a study like Framingham.

Epidemiology is the study of the occurrence of illness. Learning who is afflicted and who is spared can help provide the tools to prevent disease, even when no cure exists, and the disease process remains a mystery. This was dramatically illustrated by epidemiologist John Snow, who unearthed in 1853 a powerful clue about how to prevent cholera. He presented these figures for households supplied by two London water companies:

Water Company	Houses Served	Cholera Deaths	Rate Per 10,000
Southwark and Vauxhall	40,046	1,263	315
Lambeth	26,107	98	37

From this data Snow correctly theorized cholera could be transmitted through contaminated water, contradicting the conventional wisdom of the day that disease was generated spontaneously by mysterious vapors in the air. Snow's pioneering efforts helped fuel a public sanitation campaign that saved uncounted thousands of lives. By a similar epidemiological approach both plutonium and asbestos have been associated with lung cancer even though the specific mechanism that causes the disease remains unknown.

One of the limits, if not the hazards, of epidemiology is illustrated in another historical anecdote, possibly apocryphal, about cholera.

During the Crimean War, physicians assigned to the British Army were trying to convince the high command of the dangers of contaminated water wells in the field. One colonel, with all the flexibility and open-mindedness for which the British army was then legendary, couldn't conceive how anyone could be harmed by plain, ordinary water. He approached the well, just identified as the most dangerous to his troops' health, and scornfully drank down a dipper full of water. And of course it did him no harm whatever. Even in Snow's convincing London demonstration, ninety-seven out of one hundred households getting the contaminated water didn't have a case of cholera during his period of observation. Epidemiology is a science of probabilities. It will reveal nothing about whether a particular individual will get coronary heart disease. But it may identify specific groups in a population that are particularly vulnerable.

However, this statistical approach can provide false clues as well as valid ones. For example, heart patients were advised to avoid coffee after researchers found a positive association between coffee and coronary heart disease. The relationship was misleading. The culprit proved to be cigarette smoking, and smokers were just more likely to drink coffee.

So the Framingham study was a numbers game. The experimenters wanted to know what kinds of people got coronary heart disease and what made them different from those who did not. Did they smoke? What did they eat? Were they anxious and hard driving or confident and relaxed? There were also physical and laboratory measurements including weight, blood pressure, serum cholesterol, and the electrical activity of the heart. From these data they built a detailed portrait of coronary heart disease from a sample of 5,127 adults, of whom 404 died of coronary heart disease over the next twenty-four years.

When epidemiological studies are complete the tidy mathematical charts and tables tend to conceal the crude and approximate character of the entire exercise. And Framingham in particular was no exception. Just deciding which residents had coronary heart disease involved sig-nificant amounts of medical guesswork. The typical participant failed to appear for about one out of five physical examinations. It has been hard to keep some laboratory tests uniform over so many years. The Framingham research team was as meticulous as existing knowledge and technology permitted, but their findings, although generally con-firmed by other studies, still represented what probably happened to a small number of people, in one New England town primarily during the 1950s and 1960s.

What emerged from Framingham were a series of risk factors for coronary heart disease now familiar to most of the adult population that has ever been exposed to public service advertisements about its health. The two biggest risk factors could not be changed. Men were much more likely to develop heart disease than women, especially before age fifty-five. Pre-menopausal women were practically immune; only eleven of 1,600 such women developed coronary heart disease. The risk also increased rapidly with age. (For example, half of all coronary heart disease deaths occur in the 5 percent of the population over seventy-four years old.)

But other important risk factors looked more amenable to interven-tion. One such factor, high blood pressure, could be directly reduced by medication. Other risk factors that it appeared possible to modify included smoking, obesity, and a sedentary lifestyle.

Among the characteristics associated with a greater likelihood of coronary heart disease one drew special attention. Those with the disease tended to have higher levels of an important organic chemical called cholesterol.

Cholesterol, as most of us have been instructed, appears in large concentrations in egg yolks, in fatty beef and pork, but only in trace amounts in vegetable substances. However, most of the cholesterol in the bloodstream is manufactured by the body for a wide variety of essential purposes. Cholesterol is so important that every cell in the human body can manufacture it. The outer membrane of each cell is constructed mostly of cholesterol compounds called lipids which play a vital role in regulating what may enter and exit the cell. The body's own chemical factory, the liver, is its largest producer and consumer of cholesterol compounds. However, by weight, the heaviest concentrations of cholesterol are found in the human brain. They are even essential to the manufacture of sex hormones. It is no coincidence that when all the chemicals required to form a living creature are assembled in a hen's egg, cholesterol is a principal component.

For many years a straightforward laboratory test existed to measure the quantity of cholesterol in the blood serum, virtually all of it compounds manufactured and used by the body. The Framingham researchers found more cases of coronary heart disease among those with high levels of cholesterol in their bloodstream than among those with lower levels. Since Framingham ranks among the most frequently cited authorities for the link between cholesterol and coronary heart disease, it is revealing to examine the evidence directly. Here is an example, calculated from Framingham data at the twenty-year point:

Average Blood Cholesterol Level	Percent with Coronary Heart Disease
Low (less than 200 mg/dl)	10
Average (200–239)	12
High (240 and above)	18

(Average of 10 measurements over 20 years)

The table provides a useful vehicle for examining the strengths and the weaknesses of such relationships. On the positive side, as blood cholesterol levels rise, the upward trend in coronary heart disease is unmistakable, and other epidemiological studies have demonstrated that this relationship is robust and can be readily duplicated elsewhere.

However, the same table also shows extensive heart disease among those with low or average cholesterol levels.

Next came the most exciting part of epidemiology: Could the researchers identify groups in Framingham where the relationship between cholesterol and heart disease was even stronger and more dramatic? An answer was quickly forthcoming. The association was strongest in young and middle-aged men. If the analysis was limited to this group, those with high cholesterol were three or four times more likely to have a heart attack, chest pains, or die suddenly, compared to those with low cholesterol. And given that heart disease is the single largest cause of death, this was a relationship of indisputable importance. And enthusiasm over this relationship would fuel a scientific interest for decades to come.

Cholesterol, however, was far from a simple and universal explanation for what caused coronary heart disease. For example, high cholesterol generally did not increase the risk of coronary heart disease among women. "For women there was no relationship except in the middle decade of life," wrote Dawber, the first study director. In both men and women, beginning about age fifty, the link between high cholesterol and increased risk of coronary heart disease first weakened, and then disappeared entirely. Thus, among the elderly, the group in which most coronary heart disease deaths occur, high cholesterol did not appear to be a risk factor.

Another surprise about cholesterol emerged from Framingham, although it was never published in a scientific journal. Buried deep in a typewritten report that is almost two feet thick is a study titled "Diet and the regulation of serum cholesterol."* The Framingham researchers assumed they knew exactly why some people had higher blood cholesterol levels than others: It was their diet. To measure this link they selected 912 men and women and compared the cholesterol in their diets to the cholesterol levels in their blood. To their surprise there was no relationship. The researchers studied the intake of saturated fats, dietary cholesterol, and overall calories. None had an effect. They considered the possibility that other factors—such as differences

---

*Serum cholesterol is a laboratory measurement of cholesterol in the blood from the fluid that remains when the blood cells and clotting agents have been removed.

in physical activity—masked the effects of diet. It didn't make any difference. "There is, in short, no suggestion of any relation between diet and the subsequent development of CHD [coronary heart disease] in the study group . . . ," the researchers concluded. Furthermore, it was not lost on the Framingham team that people were already being advised to diet to lower their cholesterol, and that more elaborate campaigns were on the drawing board. They concluded with a fateful warning:

"There is a considerable range of serum cholesterol levels within the Framingham Study Group. Something explains this inter-individual variation, but it is not diet (as measured here). Clearly if there is to be an attempt to manipulate serum cholesterol level in a general population, it would be desirable to know what these powerful but unspecified forces are."

Nevertheless, among young and middle-aged men, the risk of coronary heart disease appeared to rise steadily as cholesterol levels in the blood increased. The data also showed those with a combination of risk factors were especially prone to develop coronary heart disease, and were even more vulnerable than would be expected simply by adding the individual risk factors together. It was thus that the Framingham researchers and their colleagues at the national heart institute emerged with mathematically elegant risk-factor equations for cholesterol, high blood pressure, and smoking. This was also some of the most important evidence that was on the table in 1971 when the heart institute convened a task force to plan some of the boldest and most expensive medical experiments that had ever been conducted.

• • •

IT WAS CALLED officially the Task Force on Arteriosclerosis and it would set an agenda for research on coronary heart disease that would guide the nation for fifteen years. Landmark policy decisions are made in medicine under ground rules and procedures found almost nowhere else in our society; research medicine is governed by interlocking committees of elite physicians.

Like so much of the medical world, the structure is a hierarchy of rank. On the first rung are the various primary care physicians: general practitioners, family practice specialists, and internists. The gatekeepers of the medical system must deal with such an enormous variety of human ailments that much of what they do is the application of hundreds upon hundreds of rules learned mostly by rote. Because such physicians are so often important authority figures in the eyes of patients it is often overlooked that they also are frequently following memorized rules or fixed protocols. Primary care physicians will refer the cases that cannot be dealt with by that approach to the physicians on the next level, the specialists.

When limited to a specific skill, organ, or body system, specialists can hope to know and understand a much greater fraction of the scientific literature in their field. Specialists will make more individual judgments, and their therapies may depart more frequently from what they were taught.

However, the aristocrats are the academic faculty of the medical schools and teaching hospitals. Their power reaches far beyond the fact that they may be referred the most complicated cases, and train other physicians. They decide when new therapies should now be applied on a broad scale, and determine when others should now be abandoned. The most powerful control large training and research establishments where major treatments may be tested, or some existing practice proven ineffective. More important, it is this medical elite that sits on the committees that advise the FDA on drug safety, that approve or reject multi-million dollar research grants, that appear on the expert panels at important medical meetings. Within a specialty, it is a small enough club to operate on a first-name basis.

Although a federal government agency, the heart institute interlocks tightly with this medical elite. Early in a research career, a promising academic physician may serve a tour of duty as a fellow at the heart institute. Later, the most successful academic research physicians may fill the post of institute director, or perhaps head one of the major branches. In between, the academic elite will sit on many official committees, and coauthor influential articles with institute officials. The Task Force on Arteriosclerosis that met during 1971 was one of the most important gatherings of this medical elite.

These physicians and research scientists did not win admittance to the most exclusive club in medicine by being timid thinkers, and when they sat down to plot a scientific assault on coronary heart disease, few would fault the boldness of their vision. More than twenty years of scientific research had gone into identifying the risk factors in the Framingham study. These results, by and large, fit in with other epidemiological evidence. Now they were going to go for the payoff: a scientific demonstration that enough was understood about the causes of coronary heart disease to prevent it.

Even those who harbored concerns about the ambiguity and weakness of some of the evidence could not help but be reassured by the commitment to confirming the cholesterol hypothesis through the classic scientific method. The task force remained undaunted as its various committees began the much tougher job of converting this overall mandate into detailed plans for elaborate clinical trials. They remained confident even when faced with estimates that the necessary experiments would costs millions of dollars, involve thousands of volunteer subjects, and take more than ten years. They were going to go for it, and the ink was barely dry on the report before the heart institute had endorsed the task force plan, and launched some of the most important medical experiments in history.

4
CHOLESTEROL
ON TRIAL

The medical investigators who intended to prove how to prevent coronary heart disease faced a daunting task. Clinical trials are among the most elaborate, expensive, and time-consuming forms of medical research, and these two major experiments were going to be especially difficult. The most complicated was called the Multiple Risk Factor Intervention Trial, or MR.FIT, and it still ranks as one of the largest and most demanding medical experiments performed on a group of living human beings. It took more than 10 years, involved 28 medical centers across the nation, and included 250 researchers. The costs exceeded $115 million, and just to find suitable subjects, the investigators had to examine 361,662 middle-aged men.

The first problem to be solved was an ethical dilemma that must be faced in every experiment on human subjects. The investigators had to weigh the need for knowledge about a major threat to health against the risk that trial participants might be harmed or killed.

In the most objective and convincing trials a group of people with similar medical characteristics are randomly assigned to either a treatment group or a control group. The treatment is presumed to be beneficial, or there would be no point in the trial. But the stronger the *a priori* belief that the treatment is beneficial, the more ethically troubling it becomes to deny that treatment to the control group.

Would it be proper to identify thousands of men at especially high risk for coronary heart disease, assign them to the control group, and then wait to see if the predicted number died, just for accurate comparison purposes? To resolve the problem the investigators settled on a compromise. The control group would be informed that they had an "above-average" risk of coronary heart disease, and the results of annual physical examinations from the experiment would be provided to their personal physicians. That solved the ethical problem, but the experimenters still worried that the untreated subjects were not really a true control group because each person was routinely contacted every four months, and summoned annually for a detailed physical examination. Wasn't that an intervention, all by itself? Nevertheless, the investigators elected to continue on the assumption this contact would have little or no effect over the long run.

The MR.FIT investigators' prime target was not the average American. Using the risk factor equations developed from Framingham the researchers were going to limit the experiment to a carefully selected group at highest risk from specific causes they believed they understood and could control. So they excluded the elderly, who experience most heart attacks, and young and middle-aged women, who experience few. To get the perfect 12,866 candidates at highest risk from multiple causes required examining several hundred thousand men aged thirty-five to fifty-seven. The resultant group was not exactly ready to run the Boston Marathon. Two thirds smoked cigarettes. Their typical diet included more than twice the recommended amount of cholesterol. Two out of three had developed high blood pressure early in life. Sixty percent were obese. Plainly the MR.FIT trial had met its first goal: There was plenty of risk to modify. As the trial began the men were randomly divided into two groups of equal size and similar characteristics. One group of 6,438 men was referred to the Usual Care of their physicians. The other, the Special Intervention group, became the prolonged target of a sophisticated and sustained campaign to modify their fundamental living habits.

Every clinical trial represents a series of trade-offs that determine what it can and cannot reasonably be expected to prove, and MR.FIT had a unique set of strengths and weaknesses. The tremendous appeal came because it was an objective and scientific test of the health advice already being given millions of Americans: Quit smoking, control your blood pressure, and eat less cholesterol. And it would be tested on a select group that twenty years of epidemiological research had identified as most likely to benefit from this advice. However, when and if the trial produced the predicted results, it would still leave unanswered two difficult questions. Would the same benefits accrue to a broader population not at such extraordinary risk from a particular combination of factors? After lives were demonstrably saved which risk factor should be credited for the success? Could future prevention strategy focus on cholesterol and diet, or was the combined assault the magic ingredient? There would be no way to tell, but before starting this interesting debate it was first necessary to modify the risk factors in a meaningful, measurable, and sustained manner. And that did not look easy.

It is one thing when the terrified survivor of a serious heart attack, still wearing his flimsy hospital gown, receives a stern lecture about the habits he needs to modify and the likely consequences if he does not. It is quite another to attempt such changes in a fairly ordinary middle-aged man without symptoms of ill health. Further, the physician in normal medical practice can take his best shot at influencing his patient's most dangerous habits, and consign any failures to the vagaries of human nature. Not only did the MR.FIT investigators have to achieve large, measurable behavior changes on a broad scale, they had to sustain these gains over seven years. With that challenge in mind, one of the first revisions in the study design was to drop the physician/patient model and adapt techniques more common to group therapy and behavioral psychology. The participant's principal contact with the Special Intervention group would not be a physician but a specially trained "interventionist." The early thrust of the intervention strategy would be built around ten weekly group therapy sessions during which the interventionists would seek to motivate their subjects to make far reaching changes in their daily lives. They understood that the role of the "wife or homemaker" would be critical and aimed for and achieved high levels of participation.

The interventionists' first challenge was to lower blood cholesterol through massive changes in the diet. They had to be aware that Framingham and other studies demonstrated the tenuous link between diet and the level of cholesterol in the bloodstream. However, a reasonable theory holds that diet still might work, even though the body sets a cholesterol level for itself, and manufactures an additional supply should a shortage be detected. A rough analogy would be diet and body fat. It is quite possible to have two people consuming exactly the same diet and observe that one is fat and the other is thin. In this instance food intake and body weight do not seem to be related. However, if both reduce their food consumption by 20 percent, both subjects will lose weight. Such a theory might apply to diet and serum cholesterol, although the relationship is even more indirect. The real problem is that meaningful changes in diet are extremely hard to achieve and sustain.

In the group sessions the participants were showered with information about specific foods, taught to shop for groceries, told how to order restaurant meals, even shown how to revise their favorite recipes. Participants were asked to record everything they ate and sign contracts pledging to abstain from various practices. In the best tradition of behavioral psychology participants were lavishly praised for each goal they attained. As measured by changes in eating habits the behavior modification protocol proved a huge success. The Special Intervention group cut their cholesterol intake by 42 percent. Saturated fat consumption dropped by 28 percent. And total calories fell by 21 percent. This represented a kind of dietary grand-slam home run because nutritionists still debate whether the key to dietary intervention against coronary heart disease is reducing pure cholesterol, such as egg yolks; saturated fats, such as beef and pork; or simply overall calories. The interventionists had successfully persuaded the participants to make a drastic alteration in eating habits, and sustained the changes over years, a record that any health spa or diet clinic could envy. Sadly, the enormous lifestyle changes made by the participants had little effect on the level of cholesterol in their blood. The study began with only the most modest of goals for blood cholesterol, a 10 percent reduction. The actual results were a disappointment. By one measurement method blood cholesterol dropped only 5 percent, by another 6.7 percent.

Smoking is so addictive that legend has it that even the threat of amputation of the hand did not deter tobacco use under early Persian tyrants. The interventionists' approach was considerably more subtle but more persistent, and involved an awesome variety of techniques.

Smokers got stern health lectures by physician authority figures and moving personal success stories from ex-smokers. They were offered monetary rewards—the money saved by abstaining—and were taught all kinds of tricks, such as keeping cigarettes in inaccessible places, hiding the ashtrays, and using relaxation techniques. Smokers were asked to record each cigarette they smoked and report routinely on progress or backsliding. They had "marathon groups" that spent twenty-four to thirty-six hours together while attempting not to smoke. Some centers offered four-day anti-smoking retreats. Late in the program they used hypnosis and aversion techniques. No matter what, each smoker's progress was reviewed every four months by a medical center interventionist. It's not hard to imagine that some participants might have abandoned smoking just to get the research staff off their case. At the end of four years almost half the smokers had quit entirely, an impressive result that substantially exceeded the study's target. However, they discovered that those who would benefit most—the heaviest smokers—were the least likely to quit. Nearly three quarters of the light smokers quit, compared to only one third of those with a two-pack-a-day habit.

High blood pressure was the last and simplest risk factor to attack. Except for a few of the most obese men, treatment was a matter of careful and periodic measurement of blood pressure and adjusting the medication as required. In all, 87 percent of the men were treated successfully enough to push their blood pressure below the threshold that defines moderate hypertension. Two thirds reached their specific blood pressure goal in the normal range.

The MR.FIT trial had reached a second important milestone. It had demonstrated that the behavior of a large group of men without symptoms of ill health could be successfully modified, and the changes sustained over a seven-year period. The investigators had developed methods that worked on thousands of patients in St. Louis, Los Angeles, Baltimore, Miami, and Portland. The techniques were successfully used by scores of specially trained interventionists in twenty-two clinical centers.* When all was done the evidence was abundant that the trial had changed a great many lives in an important way. That left

*The other six centers kept records, assessed electrocardiograms, and provided other support.

still to be answered the overwhelming question of how many lives had been saved.

The death watch in the MR.FIT trials was as meticulously planned as the rest of the experiment. From Framingham data the investigators developed an exact prediction—187 persons—of coronary heart disease deaths in the Usual Care group. Even after allowing for dropouts and others who wouldn't fully adhere to the program, they expected to reduce coronary heart disease deaths by more than 25 percent among those in the treatment program. A panel of three cardiologists who weren't associated with any of the centers evaluated each death to establish whether it occurred from heart disease or some other cause. Then, on the official record date of February 28, 1982, they began to tally. It was more than nine years after the experiment first began.

The trial failed completely. In overall deaths, no significant difference could be found between the two groups. In fact, slightly more total deaths occurred among the Special Intervention group. That small difference was probably a result of random chance. Focusing only on deaths from coronary heart disease did not change the picture. Out of a total of 12,866 men, the difference was only nine deaths, also probably a result of chance.

The major surprise came in the Usual Care group, the high-risk patients left to their own devices. The number of coronary heart disease deaths was 40 percent lower than expected! Even though the Usual Care group reported only minimal changes in their diet, their blood cholesterol levels declined nearly as much as the Special Intervention group, leaving only a 2 percent difference between the two. The Usual Care group didn't get a specialized anti-smoking program, but 29 percent nevertheless ceased on their own. Although fewer were treated for high blood pressure—and not as aggressively as in the Special Intervention group—the typical blood pressure in the Usual Care group was only 4 percent higher.

The investigators also faced a problem that would emerge as important in other clinical trials: The results would be clouded because the treatment had caused harm as well as benefit. Concern centered on those treated for high blood pressure in the intervention group. The medication not only lowered blood pressure, it raised blood cholesterol by 7 percent, helping to defeat one of the other trial goals. The hypertension medication also might have contributed to the deaths of some of the Special Intervention participants. The numbers were not large enough to be conclusive, but the experimenters described the indications as "ambiguous but disquieting."

The failure of MR.FIT triggered a wide range of comment and criticism in the medical community. Some treatment enthusiasts tried to explain away the failure with what might be called the Physician Conspiracy Alibi. Under this theory hundreds of ordinary physicians who happened to be taking care of a patient in the control group secretly worked to undermine MR.FIT by providing special treatment they did not give their other patients. Such malicious and unethical behavior by physicians scattered across the country seems unlikely.

The Usual Care group proved much healthier than expected, but this was likely part of the broad decline of coronary heart disease that could be observed throughout the 1970s in all age groups across the country. A second possibility was that the Framingham study substantially overstated the dangers of multiple risks.

But one fact was clear. A ten-year, $115 million research program had demonstrated that the investigators did not know nearly as much about preventing coronary heart disease as they thought they did. The health advice given to millions of Americans over decades had been tested in a large and elaborate clinical trial, and had produced no measurable benefits.

• • •

THE FAILURE OF MR.FIT did not end the scientific drive to demonstrate that coronary heart disease could be prevented. From the start many researchers believed the long-sought evidence would emerge from the classic medical intervention of drugs. However, three important requirements had to be met. First, no one had yet demonstrated it was feasible to lower blood cholesterol significantly in a free-living population for a long enough period to measure the benefits. Second, the cholesterol reductions, once achieved, must actually reduce the incidence of coronary heart disease. The investigators were searching for a risk factor that could be modified, not just a more accurate method to identify those more likely to die. Third, the treatment used to lower blood cholesterol cannot harm more people than it helps. The clearest and simplest proof is showing that lowering blood cholesterol prolongs life. Not only is a lower total mortality the main object, it is an important check against the possibility that intervention does more harm than good, perhaps reducing heart attacks but causing other unexpected problems. Those were the major challenges for a cholesterol drug trial, and the designers of the heart institute's experiment were confident that they could conquer all of them, succeeding where others had failed.

The heart institute's cholesterol drug trial was known officially as the Coronary Primary Prevention Trial, or CPPT. One of the institute's earlier steps in the assault on coronary heart disease was establishing twelve special cholesterol research laboratories called lipid research clinics. The importance of the area, and the prospect of a steady flow of federal grants, helped insure that the clinic roster included some of the biggest names in coronary medicine, including Baylor, Stanford, Johns Hopkins and the University of Washington in Seattle. The drug trial was conceived with such care that it is plain that the experimenters did not intend to become bogged down in petty bickering over research methods when the results were complete a decade later. They wanted to do everything right so that when they got the proof that they could tame coronary heart disease the evidence would be clear, convincing, and irrefutable.

The first requirement was a drug to lower blood cholesterol. From among the substances available in the early 1970s the investigators selected a drug called cholestyramine. It reduces blood cholesterol by interfering with normal digestion. The liver manufactures a substance called bile acid which circulates through the intestine where it helps break down animal fats into more usable form. When the drug, which is administered orally, is present in the intestine it binds to the bile acids, removing them from the normal pattern of circulation. Because cholestyramine is indigestible some of the bile acid is therefore excreted, prompting the liver to manufacture an additional supply. Cholesterol is one of the major raw materials needed for making bile acid, and the liver obtains much of the extra cholesterol by absorbing it from the bloodstream.

The use of this particular drug gave the experiment a biochemical purity that was absent entirely from MR.FIT's broad assault on statistical risk factors. Cholestyramine had a measurable effect on the specific cholesterol compound that was the investigators' chief suspect.

Cholesterol doesn't circulate in the bloodstream in pure form, but rather as an essential ingredient in a wide range of useful substances. The blood plasma is mostly water. Fats, both animal and vegetable, are not soluble in water. Cholesterol, with the help of other proteins, combines with fats into molecules called lipoproteins. They not only circulate through the bloodstream but also can pass through the delicate cell membranes into cells throughout the body.

Two of the most important cholesterol compounds manufactured by the human body are low-density lipoproteins, or LDL, and high-density lipoproteins, or HDL. These two key compounds, LDL and HDL, have been popularized as "bad cholesterol" and "good cholesterol." The exact role of HDL is not yet clear, but it appears to aid in the removal of cholesterol from the cells and the blood and is believed to be uniformly beneficial.

The chief culprit in coronary heart disease was believed to be low-density lipoproteins, or LDL. About 75 percent of all the cholesterol in the bloodstream is contained in LDL molecules. And the biggest specific effect of cholestyramine was to lower concentrations of LDL in the bloodstream. The investigators expected that the drug would reduce blood cholesterol by at least 25 percent, and LDL even more.

Using a drug as the means of intervention also made it feasible to improve the objectivity of the trial by making it double-blind. One half of the subjects would receive the real drug, and the other half an inert substance. Neither subjects nor experimenters would know who was getting the real drug and who received the placebo. That was the first precaution against either deliberate or unconscious bias. The involvement of twelve prestigious centers also seemed likely to increase the credibility of the research results. A separate center—at the University of North Carolina at Chapel Hill—served as referee, registry, and scorekeeper.

The investigators intended to achieve a specific result, announced and openly published in advance. Including the modest effects of diet, they expected to reduce blood cholesterol levels by an average of 28 percent in the treatment group. It would take at least three years before the lower cholesterol had any effect on coronary heart disease. By seven years' time coronary heart disease would be reduced by 50 percent in the treatment group. They insisted on a rigorous statistical test that would insure they could be 99 percent certain that the results were not a statistical fluke. "Since the time, magnitude, and cost of this study make it unlikely that it could ever be repeated, it was essential to be sure that any observed beneficial effect of lower cholesterol was a real one," the investigators explained.

What a magnificent project! The heart institute had recruited some of the finest medical researchers in the country. It would cost millions, take years, and was a classic exercise in the pure scientific method: a double-blind, impeccably objective experiment to produce a specific result predicted in advance. And what they were trying to prove was not the existence of some esoteric subatomic particle interesting only to a handful of experts. The results could benefit every man, woman, and child in the United States.

The process of locating the 3,810 perfect specimens for the trial took three full years, and required examining 480,000 middle-aged men. They searched for men with extremely high levels of blood cholesterol, higher than 95 percent of the population. In four lengthy examinations conducted over sixteen weeks, participants were scrutinized in depth. The electrical activity of their heart was recorded at rest and during exercise. The level of albumin and globulin were meticulously measured. The experimenters tested their white blood cell count, plasma glucose, and thyroid gland secretions. They accepted smokers in approximately their normal proportion in the population, but otherwise tried to keep the experiment pure by excluding those with complicating risk factors such as high blood pressure or diabetes. Participation was limited to men because in this age group their risk of heart attack is about double that of women. All the participants would go on a cholesterol-lowering diet.* In proving that they could prevent heart disease they were stacking the deck in their favor by limiting the trial participants to an unusual and specially vulnerable group. That greatly increased the odds of success in an expensive and demanding experiment. If it succeeded, questions would still remain whether the results ob-

---

*The investigators expected diet to have little effect, reducing cholesterol levels only 3–4 percent.

tained from this unusual group could be applied to the typical adult.

Even before the study began the investigators knew they had one substantial problem, but believed that they had dealt with it. In the understated words of the study design cholestyramine is an "unpleasant drug." It was, in fact, so unpleasant that the design allowed for the possibility that up to 35 percent of the participants might drop out. However, the investigators vastly underestimated how difficult it would become to induce people to take this unpleasant substance. The "harmless placebo" consisted of several scoops of finely ground sand mixed with sugar and food coloring taken before each meal. This insoluble, indigestible, and inert substance was unpleasant enough to produce moderate-to-severe gastrointestinal side effects in one out of four participants. And that was the placebo. The drug was worse. It was made of millions of tiny, chemically activated resin beads in a bulk filler. In the first year of the study 68 percent of those taking it reported moderate-to-severe side effects, the most common being constipation, gas, heartburn, and bloating. So obvious were the immediate side effects of the drug that it also affected the double-blind character of the study. By the seventh year a majority of the clinic staff and the participants correctly guessed who was taking the real drug.

The unpleasant aspects of the drug might not have been so important had it not been for one other unfortunate result. The investigators did not even come close to achieving the desired reduction in blood cholesterol. By the seventh year the cholesterol levels in the treatment group were only 6.7 percent lower than the control group. The trial design depended on achieving a difference more than four times as large. Two things accounted for the vast shortfall in cholesterol reduction. While the drug appeared to absorb bile acid effectively, the liver compensated to some extent by stepping up the manufacture of cholesterol, simply replacing some of the total removed by the drug. Second, most of the participants refused to take all six packets each day that were required to achieve the full effect of the drug. (The investigators checked on adherence by asking the subjects to return the unused packets.) So even if the cholesterol theory was absolutely correct, they had no prospect of proving it convincingly because they could not lower blood cholesterol by more than a marginal amount even under the most carefully planned clinical conditions, focusing on an ideal target population. So the second of the important, lengthy, expensive ($142 million), and elegant trials had succumbed to the very same problem: There was just not enough difference between the treatment group and the control group to prove or to disprove the hypothesis in the convincing manner the investigators had planned.

Some would conclude that the experimenters were wrong about the mechanisms of coronary heart disease. Perhaps high cholesterol was a condition frequently associated with the disease, but not a cause. If they had proved anything, the trials had demonstrated the body has a tremendously effective mechanism for maintaining blood cholesterol levels. Perhaps any intervention powerful enough to lower cholesterol substantially was predestined to do more harm than good among the general population. But the scientists who had invested much of their scientific careers trying to prove the cholesterol hypothesis would now begin to claim that these trials proved conclusively propositions that remained just intelligent, unverified theories.

It would be tempting to blame the problems of the drug trial on cholestyramine had not another trial using an entirely different drug suffered a similar fate. At the same time U.S. physicians were trying to demonstrate that coronary heart disease can be prevented, an equally ambitious effort, sponsored by the World Health Organization, was under way in three European countries. The target was blood cholesterol. The drug was called clofibrate, and the objective was to be 99 percent certain of achieving a 30 percent reduction in coronary heart disease. The prospects for achieving this conclusive evidence dimmed quickly as it became clear that clofibrate lowered blood cholesterol only 9 percent, about half the treatment effect expected. Nevertheless, the investigators led by British cardiologist Michael F. Oliver achieved one promising result. While there was no difference in the number of fatal heart attacks, significantly fewer non-fatal attacks occurred in the group taking clofibrate. But as doctors scrutinized the crucial question in all such experiments—did the treatment group live longer—the results were deeply disturbing. When the trial was halted at the end of five years the investigators reported excess deaths in the treatment group. In the group taking clofibrate, 162 deaths occurred, compared to 127 in a similar control group with equally high initial cholesterol levels.

The investigators spent years poring over the records trying to unravel why the excess deaths occurred. They documented one clear problem: Clofibrate caused gallstones "beyond a reasonable doubt." In addition, three deaths occurred during surgery to remove them. This hazardous side effect was not known when the trial began, and the evidence did not emerge until after more than two years of careful monitoring of the subjects. The remaining unexplained mortality occurred because of a variety of ailments, especially cancer, affecting the liver and digestive system. As the epidemiologist Geoffrey Rose explained: "In mass prevention each individual has usually only a small expectation of benefit, and this small benefit can be outweighed by a small risk. This happened in the World Health Organization clofibrate trial, where a cholesterol-lowering drug seems to have killed more than it saved, even though the fatal complication rate was only about 1 per 1000 per year."

Clofibrate was hardly unique in causing more harm than good in preventing coronary heart disease. The heart institute had a vast amount of clinical experience from its own Coronary Drug Project, which focused on the population at very highest risk for a heart attack—those who had already experienced one. One approach involved giving men the female sex hormone estrogen on the theory it might account for the dramatically lower heart attack rates among pre-meno-pausal women. Barely more than a year into the trial the investigators quickly abandoned large doses of estrogen when the early results showed convincingly that it caused heart attacks rather than preventing them. Three years later they discontinued more moderate doses of estrogen when no evidence emerged of efficacy "from the key end point of total mortality." While estrogen apparently did not prevent further heart attacks, it frequently caused atrophy of the testicles, reduced sex drive, breast enlargement, or impotence. The results were little more promising with a thyroid hormone called dextrothyroxine, which lowered cholesterol. It was abandoned early in the project when the trial's safety monitoring committee decided that higher mortality in the treatment group was approaching the threshold of statistical significance, and that the deaths increased steadily the longer the drug was administered. Just two drugs, clofibrate and mega-doses of the vitamin niacin, survived the full five years of the trial. Niacin looked promising in the category of non-fatal heart attacks, but it also had side effects:

92 percent reported uncomfortable flushing of the skin, 49 percent, itching, and 20 percent, other rashes. In much smaller but statistically significant numbers the niacin group reported experiencing gout, problems of the digestive system, severe scaling, and excessive darkening of the skin. There were no significant differences in critical end point of total mortality for either of the two surviving drugs. With the exception of estrogen, all the drugs in the trial were cholesterol-lowering agents.

So the recent history of drugs to prevent coronary heart disease should have provided grounds for caution as the final results of the heart institute's cholesterol drug trial were prepared for publication. This is what the CPPT investigators found, after administering cholestyramine daily to the treatment group for an average of 7.4 years:

Category	Treatment Group (1,906 Men)	Placebo Group (1,900 Men)
Deaths all causes	68	71
Coronary heart disease deaths	30	38
Non-fatal heart attacks	130	158

A literal reading of the table suggests that the effects of treatment, if there were any, were small. The results look the strongest if approached from the perspective of relative risk. While deaths from all causes number about the same, we still could say that the risk of non-fatal heart attack was "reduced by 20 percent." A second and perhaps more useful approach is to look at absolute or actual risk. From this perspective we would say 7.4 years of treatment reduced the chances of experiencing a heart attack from 8 percent to 7 percent.

These results are so meager as to raise the question of whether the cholesterol-lowering treatment had any beneficial effect. Could not these small differences be a chance result of which patients happened to be assigned to the control and treatment groups? The probability that the results occurred entirely by chance are calculated with a formula based on the number of participants and the size of the difference. Two standards are widely accepted in medical research to rule out the possibility that it was not the treatment but sheer chance that produced the result. Under the strictest standard, the experimenter wants to produce a large enough effect of treatment to be 99 percent certain the differences were not a result of chance. This was the standard proposed for the cholesterol drug trial. Under a less stringent but still widely-accepted test the experimenter wants to be 95 percent certain the effects were genuine, and not a statistical fluke. Ordinarily, results that do not meet this 95 percent confidence test are simply discarded as "not significant."*

Under either of these standards, the cholesterol drug trial was a failure because the small favorable trend in the treatment group was not statistically significant. If the fatal and non-fatal heart attacks were combined, the result got tantalizingly close to the more lenient 95 percent test, but still fell short. And when a trial fails to meet its announced statistical standards, this is the end of the matter, and it is back to the drawing boards, time to reevaluate the theory or find another approach to treatment.

However, in what was a dark day for the heart institute's long tradition of scientific excellence, events took a different turn. Over ten years time the heart institute had spent 60 percent of its $494 million budget for clinical trials on just two efforts: MR.FIT and the cholesterol drug trial. Both were bold and reasonable experiments conceived by some of the brightest minds in research medicine. By the usual standards, both had failed.

Instead of admitting the failure, the heart institute researchers went shopping for a statistical test their results might pass. Deep in the fine print of statistical theory the experimenters found a more lenient standard which their results would barely meet.†

By either a standard of common sense or more formal rules of statistical theory the trial results were at best marginal and at worst nonexistent. It was unlikely that even these minimal results could ever be duplicated in the real world of clinical practice without the ideal circumstances of a lavishly funded clinical trial. Nevertheless, the heart institute proclaimed a resounding success, perhaps borrowing the lawyers' aphorism that when the evidence is weak, argue more loudly.

The *Journal of the American Medical Association* devoted an entire

---

*In the MR.FIT trial slightly more people in the treatment group died, but the difference was so small that it was not statistically significant.
†It is called a "one-tailed" test of significance.

issue to cholesterol, and the drug trial was featured in the two lead articles. The results, the heart institute authors said, "leave little doubt of the benefit of cholestyramine therapy."

Even though the trial had been conducted only among a specially selected group of men at extremely high risk, the heart institute now sought to apply the results to a much broader population at significantly lower risk. In a conclusion that could just as easily have been an advertisement for the drug, the study report concluded:

"The trial's implications . . . could and should be extended to other age groups and women, and . . . to others with more modest elevations of cholesterol levels. The benefits that could be expected from choles-tyramine treatment are considerable." This was but the opening drum roll for what would become one of the largest medical interventions in the nation's history.

5
A DANGEROUS
CONDITION

"This is not a medically neutral term," one of the participants told the physicians and researchers who gathered at the National Institutes of Health in December of 1984. The specific word was *hypercholesterol-emia,* or in English translation, high cholesterol. "The term means there is something wrong that warrants medical attention and treatment," said DeWitt S. Goodman of Columbia University medical school.

They were about to exercise one of the most awesome powers of doctors, the power to decide who requires medical treatment and who does not. In an instant millions of Americans would acquire a dangerous condition that needed therapy under a doctor's supervision.

Officially, a special panel of fourteen persons selected by the National Heart, Lung, and Blood Institute would perform this task. They were going to assess more than thirty years of scientific research on cholesterol. This would include epidemiological studies from around the world, results from more than a dozen clinical trials, scores of animal studies, and the evidence emerging from biochemistry laboratories. After determining the relationship between cholesterol and coronary heart disease the panel would identify what portion of the American public was at risk—and estimates ranged from less than 5 percent to 100 percent of adults. Finally, having determined who was in danger, they would instruct the nation's physicians how to treat this new affliction. These conclusions would be codified in a detailed report. And they would accomplish all this in just two and a half days.

They called it a "Consensus Development Conference," and in addition to the panel was an overflow audience of more than 600 physicians and researchers. It was the largest turnout ever for such a meeting. However, the need for a "consensus conference" is a more likely sign of a major controversy in medicine than an indication that the experts now concur. Where the scientific evidence is clear, leading practitioners and researchers do not gather from all corners of the country and abroad to belabor the obvious. But the judgments once made, and however made, would carry the combined authority of the panel participants and the powerful and prestigious National Institutes of Health. They would appear in medical journals and textbooks. They would be memorized by medical students and interns. They would become a key reference cited in future scientific research. It would be an authoritative declaration from the medical elite. The panel chairman, Daniel Steinberg, a physician who worked on the cholesterol drug trial at the University of California at San Diego, expressed this with quiet medical authority:

"What we conclude here does not automatically constitute a policy statement for either the National Institutes of Health or the federal government," Steinberg said as the consensus conference began. "On the other hand it would be naive to deny our report is going to have important influence."

First, however, the panel would hear the evidence. To either the expert or novice, the growing body of evidence linking cholesterol to coronary heart disease seemed impressive. Present to describe the overall role of cholesterol was Robert I. Levy of Columbia University. Levy had initially run the cholesterol drug trial, and later headed the entire heart institute before returning to Columbia. His talk was more technical, but these were the highlights:

Levy identified low-density lipoprotein, or LDL, as the specific culprit in coronary heart disease. Measuring total cholesterol was a reasonable substitute because 60 to 75 percent of all the cholesterol compounds in the bloodstream were LDL. Furthermore, there really weren't safe and unsafe levels of LDL; the risk of coronary heart disease rose steadily as LDL rose.

Perhaps the most exciting single clue about LDL came from two Dallas researchers, Joseph L. Goldstein and Michael S. Brown, who won a Nobel prize for their work. Goldstein was present for the conference to describe his findings.

Cells, especially liver cells, have special receptors to absorb LDL from the bloodstream. The single most common genetic disorder in the United States occurs in a specific defective gene responsible for creating the LDL receptors. About one person in 500 inherits this flawed gene from one parent. As a result they have only half the normal number of receptors, extremely high levels of LDL, and are likely to experience heart attacks after age thirty. An even more catastrophic problem occurs when both parents carry the defective gene. A child who inherits two defective genes will have no LDL receptors, astronomically high levels of LDL and cholesterol, and will likely die of coronary heart disease after a few years of life. This was a narrow but crisp body of evidence linking coronary heart disease to cholesterol. A shortage of receptors left excess amounts of LDL circulating in the bloodstream, and some of the excess LDL ended up in lesions that blocked the crucial arteries supplying the heart and brain with blood. On its face, however, Goldstein and Brown's discovery undermines rather than advances the idea that too much fat and cholesterol in the diet cause coronary heart disease. High cholesterol in this instance is caused by a genetic defect, not by diet, and does not respond well to even the most aggressive diet therapy.

The panel also heard about animal experiments in rhesus monkeys and other animals in which high cholesterol diets caused the appearance of the characteristic lesions of coronary heart disease. Decreasing the cholesterol they were being fed actually caused a reduction in the size of the obstructions. But the most dramatic effects were achieved in animals that normally didn't consume meat, and had natural blood cholesterol levels far below humans. Further, the lesions were not really similar to most of those found in humans.

Under rigidly controlled conditions somewhat similar effects could be observed in human beings. For example, in experiments in mental institutions or on hospital wards, large changes in cholesterol and fat in human diet produced modest changes in the cholesterol levels in the bloodstream. But all these tidy relationships began to disintegrate when the experiment moved out of these controlled conditions into a population of healthy, free-living human beings. This was the difference between feeding mental patients fifteen egg yolks a day and conducting a clinical trial of a palatable diet among thousands of adults in their normal environment.

To many participants the pieces of the puzzle seemed to fit together to find cholesterol guilty beyond any reasonable doubt. But if the cholesterol hypothesis were true, why then had the clinical trials to confirm this hypothesis so uniformly failed? Explaining this difficulty to the consensus panel was the assignment of Richard Peto, an Oxford University epidemiologist.

"There have already been about fifteen or twenty trials, and in every trial something ridiculous happens," he said.

While no single trial was convincing, when analyzed together the trial evidence was impressive, he said. Furthermore, the greater the blood cholesterol reduction achieved, the larger the reduction in coronary heart disease. That was the broad pattern. But Peto wanted to disregard total mortality and the crucial question of whether the treatments prolonged life or shortened it.

"I don't think, in the primary prevention trials especially, that we can afford the luxury of looking at total mortality," Peto told the panel. He believed the lives that might have been saved could be too easily offset by random deaths from other causes.

The consensus conference audience included experts of scientific standing equal to those selected to present evidence, and among the first to object then was an Oxford colleague, Salim Yusif.

"Many of the trials that had the most striking effect on the reduction in cardiac deaths did not report total mortality," Yusif said. "If you include only the trials that reported total mortality the effect is actually none."

Yusif said the evidence was strong that lowering blood cholesterol indeed reduced the risk of coronary heart disease, but it was crucial to examine all the effects of treatment. When you did that the net result was zero.

The panel chairman, Steinberg, cut off Yusif in the middle of a sentence, citing a lack of time. Participants later complained that Yusif should have been allowed to complete his rebuttal. Yusif was listed on the program as a coauthor of Peto's unpublished analysis and was likely the only person present with access to the details. Other complaints came from experts in the audience who had not been invited to make official presentations.

"We simply have to acknowledge that the [trial] results have been disappointing," said Paul Meier, a University of Chicago biostatistician and frequent adviser to NIH trials. "These studies show no whisper of benefit in reducing total mortality, and I am not entirely comforted by Richard Peto's ability to explain away the significant excesses of non-coronary deaths."

Michael Oliver, the British heart expert, held a hurried conference with his British colleague, Peto. Over all the trials, the statistical trend towards increased deaths from other causes was as strong as the trend towards reduced deaths from coronary heart disease, Oliver said.

Peto, however, was trying in effect to rewrite history, because if there had been a consensus in the medical community prior to the conference, it was that no trial had yet produced convincing evidence. There was one possible exception, and it was one of the major justifications for holding the consensus conference. That trial was the heart institute's own cholesterol drug trial, which they called the CPPT, or Coronary Primary Prevention Trial. The critical task of presenting these results was reserved for a man who was playing a pivotal role in the cholesterol issue, Basil M. Rifkind. As Levy's successor he had directed the cholesterol drug trial for the heart institute. He also planned the consensus conference, selecting both the panel and speakers. He was assisted by a committee made up entirely of persons who had worked on the trial. It was Rifkind who would present what an institute official would call "the crown jewel of lipid research." As he would tell it, they had at last returned with the long-sought golden fleece, the clinical trial that proved coronary heart disease could be prevented.

"It is thought to be the first study in man to establish conclusively that lowering cholesterol reduces heart attacks and heart attack deaths," he said.

Rifkind had to explain why, despite a claimed reduction in heart attack deaths, there was no evidence that lives had been saved. Total mortality was not affected. "The conclusion of the investigators was this small discrepancy most likely reflected a chance occurrence," he said.

From the audience, the University of Chicago's Paul Meier challenged Rifkind's assessment. Expressing a conclusion that would be echoed in numerous editorials in the medical journals, Meier said:

"To call 'conclusive,' as Dr. Rifkind did, a study which showed no difference in total mortality, and by the usual statistical criteria, an entirely non-significant difference in coronary incidents, seems to me a substantial misuse of the term."

The controversies continued as the panel moved to a new subject, the role of diet. The three principal experts directly contradicted each other.

William E. Conner, an Oregon Health Sciences University diet researcher, told the panel that the best method to lower cholesterol in the blood was a stringent diet to lower cholesterol intake to about one quarter of current levels.

Scott M. Grundy, a principal author of the American Heart Association prudent diet, emphasized reducing animal fats, consigning cholesterol to a minor and secondary role.

And David Kritchevsky, a nutritionist, said both were wrong. The interactions between particular kinds of fats, fibers, and carbohydrates were so complicated that neither diet was likely to work in a free-living population where the exact ingredients of each meal could not be determined in advance. He recommended reducing the total calories in the diet, whether from animal fats, vegetables, or carbohydrates.

"We all have the same set of prepackaged data that we thaw over the fire of our own prejudices," he said.

The deeper the participants probed into the diet question the more complicated it became. If they recommended a particular diet, it was likely to affect the whole family, not just the individual at risk. That meant changing the eating habits of practically the entire country, including children. But why treat the nation's children when the buildup in the arteries did not begin until puberty in men and was extremely limited in women until menopause? And were these diets healthy for pregnant women? One member of the audience suggested that if they intended to opt for Connor's low cholesterol diet for the entire American public they had all better eat the diet first. Another said it was high time for the panel to support a vegetarian diet.

As the conference plunged forward driven by a tight schedule, as Steinberg constantly reminded the speakers, the panel began to receive more and more warnings from respected, prominent men in the field.

"After listening to the testimony today which promises so much, why don't we just hold off a bit?" asked Eliot Corday, a member of both FDA and heart institute advisory panels. "We're not ready to come out with a consensus and pour present concepts in concrete."

Robert E. Olson, a physician and specialist on nutrition at the State University of New York at Stony Brook, agreed.

"We have to keep an open mind on whether we understand this disease or not," Olson said, "My view is that we do not."

Britain's Michael Oliver warned against a rush to judgment. "As a visitor, I want to suggest you be a little cautious, that you stay within the areas where you are confident." After pointing out they had allotted only two and a half days he added:

"We approached the problem a little differently," Oliver said. "We had ten bureaucrats and we sat fifteen days over a period of two years. We spent another fifteen days writing, reading, and preparing the reports."

As Steinberg read out the final report the next morning it became clear that it was not a measured assessment of the complicated role of cholesterol in a partially understood disease. It was a campaign document and a call to action for the heart institute's cholesterol education program. It said:

"It has been established beyond a reasonable doubt that lowering definitely elevated blood cholesterol levels (specifically blood levels of low-density lipoproteins) will reduce the risk of heart attacks due to coronary heart disease."

Given three contradictory diet theories, the statement embraced them all:

"The blood cholesterol level of most Americans is undesirably high, in a large part because of our high dietary intake of calories, saturated fat, and cholesterol."

The conclusions seemed so inconsistent with the evidence that critics came to believe that the outcome was mostly decided in advance. A careful review of the proceedings yields evidence to support that claim. The course of action appeared already set, despite occasional statements that the subject was being approached with a fresh and open mind.

The comments of the heart institute's director, Claude Lenfant, are an example.

"Since the release of the CPPT we have been putting in place machinery to develop and implement a cholesterol education program," he said in prepared remarks that were read to the audience by an assistant.

Although the institute was thus committed to a cholesterol education program, Lenfant tried to assure the panel: "We have no preconceived answers to questions to be addressed."

Steinberg also wanted it both ways. "If we don't find there is a consensus," he said as the panel was about to began its private deliberations, "we'll say so. We will very humbly and with some trepidation begin work."

But a minute or two later he added that the consensus statement would be ready at 8:30 A.M. the next morning, and would be presented to the public at an already scheduled 11:30 A.M. press conference. And it turned out he was right on schedule, and in full support of the institute's cholesterol campaign.

It left some conference participants such as Edward H. Ahrens, Jr., a professor at Rockefeller University, angry to this day.

"I think the public is being hosed by the NIH and the American Heart Association," he said.

"They desire to do something good. They're hoping to God that this is the right thing to do. But they are not acting on the basis of scientific evidence, but on the basis of a plausible but untested idea."

"They have made an unconscionable exaggeration of all the data," said Thomas Chalmers, of Mt. Sinai Medical School and the Harvard School of Public Health.

So concerned about the conference conclusions were some experts from the audience, including Ahrens and Corday, that they sought to write a minority report. Their request was denied as inconsistent with with the conference's goal of "consensus."

Other NIH consensus conferences had produced illuminating summaries of complex scientific questions and were models of careful scholarship and balanced analysis. The cholesterol document, however, took this process to a new low. It reached judgments that drew outraged protests from experts in the audience and then suppressed their legitimate dissent. It relied on three unpublished studies, including Richard Peto's, and then stifled authorities who wanted to examine these new findings with greater care. The panel accepted judgments based not only on unpublished research but also untested theory, and failed to document its sources in the customary scientific manner.

It was thus that the scientific foundation was laid for the National Cholesterol Education Program. The public and the nation's physicians were next.

• • •

LIKE SOME PONDEROUS prehistoric beast, the National Cholesterol Education Program just slowly surfaced from the bureaucratic swamps at the heart institute. No pivotal or triggering event could be identified.

The program was described in surprisingly accurate detail in 1982 in a major American Heart Association policy statement. By 1983 the heart institute was conducting an expensive and detailed survey of physician and public attitudes towards cholesterol. That created the information base for a public campaign. In late 1984 the report on the cholesterol drug trial concluded with a call for a broad program. In 1985 the National Cholesterol Education Program was officially created. And in 1986 the heart institute's director first informed the advisory council of the program's existence, but rather than seeking approval, announced it as a *fait accompli*. It was officially announced to the public in 1987.

It is a program of vast scope and consequences. "A little over one out of four adults are going to be identified as needing medical attention, and needing, under supervision, to get their cholesterol lowered," said James I. Cleeman, the program coordinator. "It's a mammoth intervention and it deserves to be a mammoth intervention."

To promote this program the heart institute waged two major campaigns, one aimed at physicians, the other at the general public. Every practicing physician got a report summarizing the heart institute's "consensus" conclusions on cholesterol. A much more elaborate treatment information kit went to each of the nation's cardiologists and the 150,000 physicians in primary care, including general practitioners, internists, and family practice physicians.

As heart institute officials began to plan the selling of cholesterol it quickly became apparent that the primary obstacle was not the public but the skepticism of the nation's physicians. Fueled mainly by the highly visible and unopposed news media campaigns of the American Heart Association, the general public had been long sensitized to the alleged hazards of dietary cholesterol, and the heart institute's opinion polls reflected the tremendous impact of years of media campaigning. In 1983, two thirds of the public believed a high-fat diet had a large effect on coronary heart disease, and nearly as many believed dietary cholesterol an equally important hazard.

A majority of the nation's physicians disagreed, the heart institute learned. While nine out of ten thought smoking had a large health effect, only 28 percent were equally concerned about a high-fat diet, and only 39 percent about elevated blood cholesterol.

Therefore, the nation's doctors, not the public, became the first public relations target of the heart institute. Even the slogan that emerged later would exploit the discovery that the public had been more readily convinced about cholesterol than the doctors who had to deal with heart disease every day. "Ask your doctor about cholesterol" was the message on a heart institute poster.

The public was also largely unaware that a lively debate was being waged mostly out of view in the nation's medical journals and scientific meetings, and that expert opinion was never unanimous. In 1980, for example, no less than the American Heart Association's own president, Thomas N. James, had dissented on diet.

"I wish to present some personal reservations about our nonexceptional advice, which is taken by the public as meaning everyone should be concerned about their dietary cholesterol," said James in a broad critique of emphasis on diet delivered to the association's annual scientific meeting. His views were reported in the American Heart Association's own medical journal, *Circulation*, with the disclaimer that this was not necessarily the heart association position.

The heart institute's director, Claude Lenfant, encountered stiff resistance from his own Advisory Council, a panel of influential physicians who advise on and approve research. Lenfant never asked this panel to approve a National Cholesterol Education Program since it was "public education" and not medical research. But he did have to ask them to approve money for a research project to learn how most effectively to influence the nation's physicians about cholesterol, especially on the diet question.

In a gathering noted for the calm and well-modulated tone of its proceedings, a heated debate ensued, and in a rare rebellion the panel refused to endorse the director's proposal.

"Physicians just aren't convinced [about cholesterol]," said panel member Eliot Corday, who led the dissent.

But despite such reverses, the heart institute's machinery cranked relentlessly on. Six months later, the proposal was resubmitted and rejected again after another debate. But after another year, at a moment when the mix of panel attendees was slightly different, a scaled-down research program was narrowly approved.

"I must admit that each time we have a discussion about cholesterol it's interesting," said Lenfant, his victory at last in hand. And the main reason for the relatively low public profile of the National Cholesterol Education Program is that its first goal was influencing the physician community.

The heart institute's eager partners in promoting cholesterol consciousness are the drug companies, which are understandably excited that the government is creating the largest new market in decades. Most drugs face the inherent limitation of effectiveness—they soon solve the medical problem for which they were intended, and are no longer necessary. The biggest money-makers are drugs needed indefinitely. This places cholesterol treatment in the select group of mega-drugs: tranquilizers, hypertension, and angina medication. As a consequence the medical journals were soon packed with advertisements for cholesterol-lowering drugs, and salesmen were knocking on the doors of physicians' offices from coast to coast. And what could be more effective in beating down sales resistance and physician skepticism than the explicit endorsement of government experts? Therefore drug company advertising literature would frequently cite the National Cholesterol Education Program.

In late 1988 this already powerful combine acquired important new partners. The American Medical Association, a major drug company, and two food companies with low-cholesterol products joined forces to launch a massive campaign that reached the public beginning early in 1989. It included national and local television programs, special magazine features, cereal box advertisements, cholesterol books, videocassettes, brochures, discount coupons, posters, and study guides for physicians.

This, however, was not exactly a public service campaign, but a business scheme to sell physicians' services and other products. In announcing the promotional scheme to the nation's physicians, the AMA said:

"The AMA's Campaign Against Cholesterol will use national and local television to tell the public about the risks of high blood cholesterol and *the availability of cholesterol testing through your office* [emphasis added]. The second sponsor, Merck Sharp & Dohme, was already aggressively marketing its new cholesterol-lowering drug, lovastatin. Kellogg would launch a new oat cereal, and American Home Products would promote a cooking oil spray that, like almost all vegetable oils, contained no cholesterol. The National Cholesterol Education Program guidelines provided that treatment should not begin without a complete physical examination, a patient history, and laboratory workup. This was not lost on the AMA, which noted pointedly that screening programs had found "as many as 25 percent of the participants either have no personal physician, or have not seen their doctor within the past five years." Thus a program that may have begun as sincere but misdirected zeal for the public good became intertwined with greed. The world was learning how much money could be made scaring people about their cholesterol. And it was already clear that these mainstream organizations were being joined by thousands of less responsible profiteers offering miracle treatments, wondrous diets, cholesterol checkups, and a variety of other wares with benefits that were non-existent, unproven, or just plain hazardous.

One fact was therefore certain: The American public and the physician community would receive a hard sell on the dangers of cholesterol, an effort sure to drive people by the millions into the National Cholesterol Education Program.

While the avalanche of information reaching the public uniformly emphasized the dangers of cholesterol, questions continued to be raised in the nation's medical journals. Since 1985, when the campaign was created, critical articles or editorials have appeared in the following important publications: *Annals of Internal Medicine, Mayo Clinic Proceedings,* the *Journal of the American Medical Association, Medical Care, Circulation,* and the *Journal of the American College of Cardiology.*

While this stream of medical literature guaranteed that balanced information was available to the inquiring medical researcher, the cholesterol opponents still seemed to lose ground. They were individuals who conducted research or wrote an analysis and that was the end of it. Opponents had no money to sponsor national conferences. Their articles weren't mailed to the nation's medical writers along with press releases. Unlike the heart institute, they had no means to build a massive alliance of parties with a financial or other stake in the cholesterol question. They didn't have opinion polls and research grants to teach them how to select target audiences and influence them most effectively. And given that the heart institute is the principal and most important source of funds for research, it is a tribute to the independence of the medical community that so many physicians spoke out, and that the journals featured their views so prominently and in such detail. But opponents lacked the money, skills, and perhaps even the interest to take their case to the general public.

So thus far they have been overwhelmed by the public extravaganza launched not just by the heart institute, but by a growing coalition that resembles a medical version of the military-industrial complex.

First are the "authorities"—the experts in the medical schools—most of whom head or are involved with one of the twelve lipid research laboratories that the heart institute established twenty years ago for the big clinical trials. Most of these researchers have devoted many years of their careers as principal investigators in the MR.FIT and the cholesterol drug trial, neither one of which produced evidence that lives were saved. Furthermore, these large research establishments rely heavily on heart institute funding. Most of the rest of the money comes from drug companies with cholesterol-lowering drugs.

Next is the heart institute itself. Could the political potential of making every American aware of his cholesterol level have been lost on the heart institute? Put another way, is it possible to imagine a more effective scheme to raise its public profile any higher?

The heart institute, in turn, is tied closely to the drug industry. Not only does it frequently test promising new drugs without charge to the companies, it is not bashful about publicly endorsing specific products it deems useful. The closeness of this relationship was driven home one day when I called the office at the heart institute responsible for cholesterol research, seeking some information, and giving my name, but no title.

"And what drug company do you represent?" asked the secretary.

And last, but not least, comes the American Heart Association, which had long urged just such a cholesterol campaign.

Here is a combine of awesome power and reach. It boasts the authority of the federal government, the money and the sales force of the drug companies, the clout of the AMA, the reach and reputation of the American Heart Association. To make matters simpler, the entire establishment is controlled by an interlocking directorate.

For example, Robert I. Levy was a lipid expert at Columbia University, then helped launch the major trials at the heart institute; next he directed the entire heart institute, and now heads the research subsidiary of a drug company, Sandoz Pharmaceuticals. When the consensus conference needed an expert to present an overview of the cholesterol problem, it invited Levy.

Daniel Steinberg is a physician and cholesterol researcher who headed the lipid research laboratory at the University of California at San Diego. He was also a principal investigator for the heart institute's cholesterol drug trial, and then served on the panel that developed the specific details of the National Cholesterol Education Program. But his key role was as chairman of the Consensus Development Conference panel in 1984.

That conference also heard from a cholesterol specialist named Antonio Gotto. Gotto also happened to be president of the American Heart Association, which was pushing for a campaign. He was also head of the Baylor University lipid research laboratory and worked on the cholesterol drug trial.

For years the American Heart Association's leading diet expert was a Dallas cholesterol researcher named Scott M. Grundy. The consensus conference heard him as a main speaker on diet. And Grundy also chaired the subcommittee that drew up the diet provisions of the National Cholesterol Education Program. And his laboratory at the University of Texas has also tested cholesterol-lowering drugs.

In November of 1988 the heart institute sponsored a national conference on cholesterol, and the chairman was John LaRosa. LaRosa heads the lipid laboratory at George Washington University. He also chairs the diet committee of the American Heart Association. He invested years as an investigator in the heart institute's cholesterol drug trial.

When Merck introduced a new cholesterol-lowering drug called lovastatin the whole apparatus went into action. For reporters who might want an intimate local flavor Merck helpfully provided the names and telephone numbers of nearby research physicians who would talk about the drug and identify patients, presumably for personal testimonials.

It is likely that one reason these important physicians consented to such an arrangement is because their laboratories are heavily involved in research funded by Merck. Thus the Merck press release shows that in Houston a reporter might call Antonio Gotto. In Washington, the company suggests contacting John LaRosa, in Dallas, Scott M. Grundy, and in San Diego, Daniel Steinberg.

There is no reason to doubt the honesty, sincerity, and expertise of any of these men, or a dozen others with multiple roles in the cholesterol establishment. The terrible danger of such a closed loop is that important and basic questions are neither asked nor answered. And that is exactly the problem that occurred when a panel of lipid researchers and heart institute officials designed the National Cholesterol Education Program. To observe those shortcomings consider how the program will work from the patient's eye view.

...

BY SWEEPING DECREE, the National Cholesterol Education Program divides the American public into three groups:

Those with serum cholesterol levels of 240 mg/dl or above have "high blood cholesterol" and require treatment under medical supervision for the rest of their lives. There is no quantum leap in risk at this cutpoint; it was arbitrarily selected to target 25 percent of the adult population.

Next come those with "borderline-high" cholesterol, defined as levels from 200 to 239 mg/dl. In this group, men with one additional risk factor and women with two will require medical treatment.* The intent of the program's designers to use fear as a weapon can be seen in the decision to label as "borderline-high" cholesterol what is actually average cholesterol.

Finally those below 200 mg/dl have "desirable" cholesterol levels. Individuals in this group are to be released with a lecture or brochure about the dangers of cholesterol, and retested every five years.

Considering that treatment may prove unpleasant, inconvenient, expensive, or all three, it is obviously important to identify correctly those likely to reap some benefit, to classify people into the correct group. Further, a program that falsely reassures those with substantial risk is a dangerous one, perhaps worse than no program at all. Nevertheless, the panel that designed the National Cholesterol Education Program knew that it would result in the treatment of millions of people classified into the wrong cholesterol group.

Poor performance by clinical laboratories accounts for part of the problem. The heart institute's twelve lipid research laboratories proved that serum cholesterol can be measured accurately. A careful series of tests revealed an average error of 1 to 2 percent. Furthermore, all twelve laboratories could be calibrated to the same reference sample. This is a crucial step because one key danger of these devices is a large and

---

*Additional risk factors include smoking, obesity, diabetes, high blood pressure, family history of heart disease, other vascular disease, and low levels of HDL.

consistent upward or downward bias for all samples. Although it would result in some misclassification, a 3 percent error rate is both realistic and would confine the errors to borderline cases. And this, in fact, was the final target set by the program's laboratory standards panel.*

Unfortunately, hardly any clinical laboratories meet this standard. For example, the College of American Pathologists surveyed a group of laboratories, and found the error rate was, on the average, 6.2 percent. A 1988 survey showed that one out of five clinical laboratories had an error rate of 9 percent or more. And these are the good laboratories, the 5,000 who are voluntary members of a quality assurance program of the College of American Pathologists. Three quarters of the major clinical laboratories are not members. And the measurement quality in the 30,000 mom and pop laboratories in doctors' offices and group practices is just anyone's wild guess.

How serious is a 9 percent average error rate? Taking into account that some errors will be smaller and others larger than average, we can say that in 95 percent of the cases individuals with about average cholesterol, or 220 mg/dl, could expect readings that would vary from 187, or deep in the "desirable" category, all the way to 267, or far into the treatment group.

Consider the experience of Walt Bogdanich, a *Wall Street Journal* reporter who sent a blood sample to five different New York laboratories. He got back results that would have placed him in the high, borderline, and low cholesterol groups.

When the samples of 117 Tennessee state employees were sent to a commercial laboratory, 75 percent fell into the treatment group. Independent tests showed only 25 percent should have been so classified. The biggest reason for the discrepancy: The laboratory equipment inadvertently inflated all the readings by approximately 6 percent.

These weaknesses were well known to the framers of the National Cholesterol Education Program; most of the facts are taken from a report prepared for the heart institute. This is the response of Basil M. Rifkind, the research physician who heads the cholesterol research branch for the heart institute:

---

*As an interim goal the panel suggested a 5 percent error rate standard, which would misclassify approximately one out of three in a single measurement.

"This is by no means a good answer, but a lot of medicine is conducted these days in other areas where measurement is less than optimum. Holding back until you're really satisfied would just slow things down tremendously."

Unfortunately, sloppy laboratory work is not the only problem in accurately identifying the right people for treatment. An individual's serum cholesterol levels are not stable. The most detailed report on the problem comes from D. M. Hegsted of Harvard University. He found a 5 to 9 percent variation in serum cholesterol levels, even among institutionalized individuals on a uniform diet. He estimated that a single measurement would result in misclassification of one out of three persons tested. The heart institute panel's recommendation for at least two cholesterol measurements prior to beginning medical treatment helps this situation somewhat. But it has no effect on the single biggest source of inaccurate readings: systematic bias by uncalibrated laboratory machines.

The most inexplicable of all decisions in the measurement area occurred when the adult treatment panel elected to base the threshold for drug therapy on LDL, or low-density lipoprotein. The single most important public health decision in the National Cholesterol Education Program involved how many millions of people will be placed on a lifetime regimen of cholesterol-lowering drugs, and at what level of risk for coronary heart disease. Rather than using a simple and widely understood serum cholesterol measurement, the panel decided to set a level of LDL at 190 mg/dl.

The problems of measuring serum cholesterol are minor in comparison to getting an accurate fix on LDL. Laboratory tests for LDL are not generally available. Therefore the panel recommended that physicians deduce the level of LDL using a formula whose key component was HDL, or high-density lipoprotein. While HDL can be measured, the quantities are so much smaller that the error rate is extremely high.

"Often, [HDL] plasma high-density lipoprotein cholesterol measurements lack sufficient accuracy to be of practical use in an individual clinical setting," concluded a group of researchers from Stanford in the *Journal of the American Medical Association.* Another survey found in

39 percent of the labs checked the average error exceeded 31 percent. The fact that HDL levels vary independently of LDL adds still another source of error.

The failures of the National Cholesterol Education Program grow more severe as the patient moves from classification to medical treatment. The initial approach calls for a cholesterol-lowering diet of moderate severity, with laboratory tests at six weeks and three months to determine the results achieved. If little change occurs, a more severe diet is imposed. The principal effect of this therapy will be to subject twenty-five million adults and their families to a sample of the inconvenience, frustration, and failure that medical scientists experienced exploring the link between diet and heart disease.

Many observers in the medical community were surprised to discover that the heart institute had made diet the front line treatment since it had abandoned diet as a prevention strategy sixteen years earlier. Back in 1971 the heart institute had rejected an elaborate proposal for a clinical trial based on diet alone, concluding the effects were so small that it would take an experiment with 100,000 people to produce a measurable effect, and even then it might fail. Given the extensive scientific record on the question, it is remarkable indeed to find dietary intervention once again the center of medical and public attention. The record is replete with evidence that the link between diet and heart disease is weak, and efforts to alter serum cholesterol with diet are maddeningly complicated and fraught with considerable peril. Here is what the research shows:

The Framingham study, which showed no relationship between the diet and serum cholesterol levels, meant that those with high serum cholesterol levels might well have low cholesterol diets. And some of those with low levels were gorging themselves on eggs and meat. However, it was still possible that a high fat and cholesterol diet might increase the risk of a heart attack, if studied across a broader range of dietary habits. And soon that question was the target of an elaborate heart institute research study.

The diets of 16,349 men in Framingham, Puerto Rico, and Honolulu were examined, and the subjects were followed for six years. Then the diets of those who had experienced heart attacks were compared with those who were still free of coronary heart disease. There was no difference in cholesterol in the diets of the two groups. There was also no difference in consumption of saturated fats or total calories from food. And these similarities were found in all three different geographic areas.

Only one dietary difference emerged, and it could be found in all three locations. Alcohol consumption was 33 to 100 percent higher in those free of coronary heart disease. William P. Castelli, the current director of the Framingham study, found the likely reason for the effect of alcohol in a separate project: Alcohol raises HDL, or so-called "good cholesterol." It is possible to imagine the frustration experienced by diet researchers upon this discovery. (Heart researchers spend years studying heart disease and emerge with the advice: Have another drink.)

"If the cross-sectional correlations among Japanese men in Honolulu and San Francisco could be translated into intervention results," said Castelli, "a non-drinker who began drinking five ounces of alcohol a week would accomplish as large a reduction of LDL cholesterol as he would by the usually suggested lipid-lowering diets."

Castelli hastened to add he was not serious. "This is not, and should not be taken as a prescription for altering blood lipids by increasing alcohol intake. On the contrary it is a warning against too hasty modification of dietary habits on the basis of limited and poorly understood evidence." These studies came quite late in the game, as far as diet was concerned, being published in 1977 and 1981. The deeply held belief in the role of diet had roots in earlier research that had such an enormous impact that it needs to be included in any serious discussion of diet and heart disease.

It was called Coronary Heart Disease in Seven Countries and it was led by one of the most energetic and prolific figures in heart research, Ancel Keys of the University of Minnesota. He studied Japanese farmers and Finnish factory workers, Italian peasants and U.S. railroad employees, Dutch shopkeepers and Yugoslavian food processing workers. When Keys put all the data together he had a striking chart in which a nation's coronary heart disease rate appeared to march upward in lock step with the typical amount of saturated fat in that population's diet. In Japan, for example, both the consumption of animal fat and the incidence of coronary heart disease were a fraction of the United States.

So how are the two apparently conflicting findings on diet to be reconciled? Among the residents of Framingham, Massachusetts, no link can be detected between the cholesterol in their diets and either their blood cholesterol levels or their chances of suffering a heart attack. But taken as a group, the Framingham residents consume more animal fat and also experience higher levels of heart disease than their Japanese counterparts, taken together.

An important lesson can be learned from the resolution of similar contradictions about salt and high blood pressure. The human body has a powerful mechanism to maintain a specific level of dissolved salt and quickly eliminates any surplus. Therefore normal adult consumption can vary over an extremely wide range without altering the internal balance, just as differences in dietary fat and cholesterol intake do not much affect blood cholesterol levels. But if the internal levels of dissolved salt do become excessive one response is to increase the total fluid volume in the body, and this can quickly lead to elevated blood pressure. Researchers also discovered that some countries, particularly certain underdeveloped nations, had diets that included much less salt. And these countries also had a much lower incidence of high blood pressure. Since the American diet included far more salt than biologically necessary, health authorities launched a vast campaign to get the nation to cut down on salt.

Nearly two decades after limiting salt became synonymous with healthy living the relationship was convincingly demonstrated to be mostly a mirage. A major international research project in 32 nations showed that while the incidence of hypertension varied widely, salt intake had little to do with it. Only if salt was almost totally eliminated from the diet was there a useful effect. The lifestyles and habits of millions of Americans had been changed to little or no purpose.

Where did the research go wrong? Comparisons between countries can be particularly treacherous, noted William Ira Bennett, a physician and editor of the *Harvard Medical School Health Letter*. "This is a tricky business," he said, "because you can bet that differences in salt intake are not the only differences between two countries." Furthermore, the researchers initially did not measure dietary salt accurately enough and did not study enough countries.

So great are similarities between the salt and cholesterol questions it is likely that the international comparisons of cholesterol are also misleading except at the extremes. Should not comparisons involving thousands of similar people in one community provide a more realistic measure than a single comparison between two dissimilar countries? Just as in the case of salt, the enduring lesson of international studies may ultimately be to show that only at extreme values, such as a diet almost entirely free of animal fat and cholesterol, does consumption have a useful effect for most individuals.*

Partly as a practical accommodation to the American palate, more moderate cholesterol-lowering diets were developed in an attempt to prevent heart disease. However, this leaves a diet that is less likely to be hazardous but also unlikely to be effective. And that is the problem that millions of Americans will face when placed on a medically supervised diet. And again, careful scientific studies document the meager results that are likely to occur.

The reports are legion, and the results are numbingly familiar. An approach to dietary intervention is developed, and it is tested among a handful of subjects with a totally controlled diet under institutional conditions. These are called metabolic ward studies. On a short-term basis serum cholesterol is frequently lowered on the order of 15 to 20 percent. And metabolic ward studies exist for a large number of approaches, including high polyunsaturated fat diets, low saturated fat diets, monosaturated fat (olive oil) diets, zero cholesterol diets, and vegetarian diets. However, responsible scientific researchers know the only way to measure the effect of a diet intended for millions of free-living individuals is to test it among a large number of people in a normal lifestyle. And when cholesterol-lowering diets are thus tested the promising results mostly disappear.

• • •

---

*On the other hand, since the western diet already contains more saturated fat and salt than needed, moderation remains sensible advice.

Here is a table of large experiments on diet:

Trial	Year	Participants	Length	Percent Cholesterol Lowering
Heart-Diet Pilot	1968	962	7 months	10.5
MR.FIT	1984	6,428	7.5 years	6.7
Northwestern*	1986	220	6 weeks	5.2
CPPT (diet only)	1984	3,806	7.4 years	3.8

*The Northwestern experiment had a second phase to test the effects of oat bran. It appeared to reduce cholesterol further, but the results were too small to reach statistical significance. Despite enormous public interest in oat bran, this seems to be the only sizable study among free-living individuals.

These trials had different numbers of participants at different initial cholesterol levels. The severity of the diets varied as did the length of the experiments. But the results are surprisingly uniform, and describe the likely results of a cholesterol-lowering diet with good to excellent adherence. Both the Northwestern and MR.FIT investigators expressed disappointment that they achieved only about half the cholesterol lowering achieved in the much older Heart-Diet Pilot, whose results they hoped to duplicate.

However, the average figures above conceal the widely varied response of individuals. The Heart-Diet Pilot provided the most detailed insights into individual variability. For one quarter of all individuals, diet has little or no effect. But about one out of seven prove to be diet responders, and experience cholesterol lowering equal to or greater than the best results in the table.* Thus those with a weak dietary response could expect cholesterol lowering of 3.8 percent or less; the lucky diet responders, 10 percent or more; and the remaining majority about 5 to 6 percent. If the evidence is absolutely clear on one question, it is that diet offers no short-term benefits; to produce a measurable effect on the risk of a heart attack would require adherence for from five to twenty years.

These facts had to be familiar to the physicians who developed the adult treatment guidelines for the National Cholesterol Education

*Anecdotal stories of dramatic changes from diet likely come from rare diet responders, poor laboratory measurement, normal individual variation, or some combination of the three.

Program. Not only are these the major studies from the scientific literature, many of the panel members were principal investigators for the two largest trials, MR.FIT and the CPPT. A careful reading of the program's treatment guidelines for physicians reveals repeated endorsement of the benefits of diet intervention, but a curious silence about what specific results may be expected. In fact, the single expected result cited came from a ward metabolic study which was not identified and claimed reductions two to four times higher than what the heart institute actually achieved in major trials.

Equally curious was the decision to enforce diet through medical supervision. Some doctors might like the extra business, but few were equipped or trained for detailed dietary counselling and follow-up that are essential to achieve any results at all. Finally, adding a pseudo-scientific veneer to the whole exercise by measuring the results with inaccurate cholesterol tests would add a whole new dimension that would vary from confusion to failure. (Gee, Mr. Jones, what a dramatic drop in your cholesterol. Well, doctor, it must be all those extra eggs I've been eating.)

The final component of the program was to recommend that millions of Americans undertake a life-long regimen of an expensive and unpleasant drug that the heart institute's own elaborate tests showed had at best marginal effect and possibly none. "The drug of choice," according to the program treatment guidelines, is cholestyramine or the chemically similar colestipol. James I. Cleeman, the program coordinator, estimated that one out of five referred for treatment would ultimately be placed on drug therapy. Early reports at the American Heart Association meeting in November 1988 suggested Cleeman's estimate was proving accurate: In one Iowa community 19.4 percent were placed on drugs, in another, 18.7 percent.

The benefits of cholestyramine were explored in detail earlier: Giving the drug for 7.4 years to 1,906 men at extremely high risk for a heart attack had produced no effect on life expectancy, but a favorable trend towards fewer heart attacks, a benefit too small to pass the usual scientific tests of validity. Given such meager benefits, what about the costs? Even ignoring the possibility that some of the cholestyramine trial results occurred partly by chance, the figures are so surprising it is a wonder the heart institute even considered the idea. A total of $23 million in drugs, administered for 14,250 person-years may have prevented 36 heart attacks, or $647,205 per heart attack.*

Since the heart institute now proposes to give cholestyramine to those at lower risk than the specially selected trial participants, the above figures exaggerate the benefits. And while different approaches to cost benefit analysis may produce somewhat different results, the remarkable fact was that the heart institute steadfastly refused to consider the cost question in any way.

The cost issue was first raised back at the consensus conference in 1984. Robert I. Levy, who headed the agency for many years, cut off a discussion about cost at the consensus conference with this statement:

"When you think about costs, think about the fact that coronary artery disease is costing sixty billion dollars. So how much is worthwhile for relieving those costs?"

Daniel Steinberg, the consensus panel chairman, said, "I don't think we're trying to focus here on the costs. I think we're here to decide what is in the best interests of the health of the nation. We'll let some other people at some other conference work that out."

But Steinberg didn't work the problem out when he became a member of the panel that designed the treatment guidelines for the program, and in fact no one at the heart institute seems to have addressed the cost question. The program's current coordinator, Cleeman, said not only would it be difficult to estimate the costs and benefits, it would be "inappropriate."

And what might those costs be? The most expensive component is the drug therapy. Giving cholestyramine to five million people would cost, at current retail prices, approximately ten billion dollars a year.† The program should generate thirty to one hundred million doctors' office visits a year, and perhaps one hundred million laboratory tests for cholesterol levels. Before treatment begins the program recommends

---

*The drug costs are adjusted downward because the drug was so unpleasant that 35 percent of the prescribed doses were not taken.

†Some competing cholesterol-lowering drugs are cheaper, others are more expensive.

a complete physical examination, patient history, and laboratory workup. Since a significant amount of screening will occur at routine physical checkups, not all the exams can be considered additional costs. But treatment by diet alone would entail three additional doctor's office visits per year, or seventy-five million visits. Thus the cost of laboratory tests and physician services should total three to ten billion dollars. Therefore it seems conservative to estimate that the National Cholesterol Education Program will cost society from ten to twenty billion dollars a year.

This amount is equivalent to the total federal nutritional assistance to the poor, including food stamps. It is roughly the same as the all federal programs to build and improve highways. It is two to three times the total cost of space flight and exploration.

When I raised these comparisons with a member of the panel that developed the program guidelines, he objected to comparing the indirect costs of the cholesterol program with direct federal spending programs involving public money.

In fact, however, the enormous costs of the National Cholesterol Education Program are more insidious. In an age of soaring deficits a ten- to twenty-billion-dollar new federal program would face intense critical scrutiny, and would have to survive severe competition with other pressing national needs. The costs of this program are no less real. They are just better concealed. But the money for this effort will be collected on the authority of doctors, primarily for the benefit of drug companies, in a scheme engineered by a small group of men and women who mistakenly believed they were doing something good.

6
THE DANGERS OF
LOW CHOLESTEROL

In scientific research as in life people tend to find what they are looking for, to see what they expect to see. It is a powerful truth indeed that reveals itself unasked, and one such case featured an internationally famous, all-star cast of cholesterol researchers. The discovery was not only surprising, it was an ugly and uninvited complication to the cholesterol problem.

These were the biggest guns in the epidemiology of coronary heart disease. From Britain came Geoffrey Rose, a world authority. William B. Kannel of Boston University, the second director of the Framingham study, was on the research team. It included Ancel Keys of the University of Minnesota, who had led the massive seven-countries study. The team had an excellent reason to believe that the culprit cholesterol was going to be found guilty of a second crime, an association with higher rates of colon cancer.

With the same logic applied to the seven-countries study—comparing entire nations rather than individuals—the team had found a striking relationship. The data already seemed to show that countries with more saturated fat in their diets had more coronary heart disease. Next came the discovery that countries with more coronary heart disease also had higher rates of colon cancer. All that remained to close the net tightly around the culprit was to demonstrate that the individuals who got colon cancer also had high cholesterol levels. To show that high blood cholesterol levels were responsible for not just one major hazard to life but two would be an important achievement. The year was 1974.

So the team collected every colon cancer case it could find among the participants in six big epidemiological studies, including Ancel Keys's seven countries, Kannel's Framingham men, English businessmen, and American Western Electric Co. employees. Then they examined the serum cholesterol levels of the colon cancer victims.

The men with cancer did not have high cholesterol levels as expected. They had the opposite. A strong and consistent trend showed the cancer victims had lower-than-average cholesterol levels compared to others in their community or country. A baffled group of researchers suggested that this needed further study and suggested, among other things, a fresh look at polyunsaturated fats. They had good reason to look at vegetable oils. A few years before, in 1971, Morton Lee Pearce and Seymour Dayton had reported in *Lancet* an excess of cancer deaths in a diet trial using diets high in polyunsaturated fats. In an action that was to be repeated many times, the pro-cholesterol researchers published a rebuttal saying that Dayton and Pierce's results were likely a result of random chance. Any unwelcome findings were quickly dismissed as probably a statistical fluke.

However, the same relationship between lower cholesterol and cancer was found again in 1978 in the World Health Organization's massive trial of the drug clofibrate. So many cancer cases occurred in the treatment group that it outstripped any beneficial or protective effect of the cholesterol lowering. However, the findings raised more questions than they answered. Was it the drug or the cholesterol lowering itself that caused the cancer? The weight of expert opinion favored blaming the drug. Other smaller studies began to appear linking low cholesterol to cancer, but the authors usually dismissed the finding as a "pre-clinical" indication of cancer, a matter of no great importance.

By 1980 French researchers had found the same relationship in a study of 7,603 male government employees. The risk of cancer began to climb steadily as cholesterol levels fell below 200 mg/dl, the level the heart institute today calls "desirable." The French findings did not suggest that high cholesterol had any protective effect against cancer. But cancer incidence rates climbed unmistakably as levels fell below 200. Even though the low cholesterol levels were measured as early as seven years before the onset of cancer, the French researchers accepted the prevailing view this was not likely to be a causal link, "but in all probability reflects the advance of the clinical course of cancer."

So many investigators had found the low cholesterol/cancer association that epidemiological researchers began to test the customary explanation that a drop in cholesterol levels was merely a "pre-clinical" indicator of cancer, a byproduct of cancer that could not yet be detected.

In an analysis for the *Journal of the National Cancer Institute* Paul D. Sorlie and Manning Feinleib went back to the Framingham data. They reported "in some cancer cases the serum cholesterol level was lower than that expected as much as sixteen to eighteen years before cancer diagnosis." That made low cholesterol almost as powerful a predictor of cancer as high cholesterol was of coronary heart disease. They did not, however, regard their analysis as conclusive.

Next, researchers at the National Cancer Institute measured the same relationship in a much larger group of Americans, 12,488 men and women who participated in the National Health and Nutrition Examination Survey. This was a bigger, more recent, and more representative sample of the American population than Framingham. The men with the lowest cholesterol levels were more than twice as likely to be diagnosed with cancer than those with the highest cholesterol levels. Further, the longer the follow-up, the stronger the relationship. They also found a similar relationship among women, but it was much weaker. "It may be premature to dismiss the inverse relationship between serum cholesterol and cancer simply as a pre-clinical marker of disease," the authors wrote in *Lancet*.

The relationship between low serum cholesterol and cancer remains unclear, and the statistical association found in so many studies neither proves nor disproves a causal link. But it also seems clear that this was an unwelcome finding to many researchers, who exercised an extraordinary caution that could not be found when they discussed the relationship between high cholesterol and heart disease. It is not, however, difficult to find a theory to explain the cancer link. The gatekeepers of the human body, the cell membranes, are composed of cholesterol compounds called lipids. As the British heart researcher, Michael F. Oliver, put it:

"A key question that I asked six years ago remains unanswered: How much cholesterol can be depleted from cell membranes over many years without alteration of their function?" In other words, at what point and how did the membrane function become sufficiently compromised to admit carcinogens?

Two other hazards of low cholesterol remain less understood and are even more poorly documented. Low cholesterol levels are associated with both gallstones and stroke.

The evidence on gallstones emerged from two specific cholesterol-lowering trials, one dietary and one drug. Many years after the end of a Veterans Administration diet trial, the autopsy records of the deceased participants were examined. Those on the high polyunsaturated diet were about twice as likely to have gallstones as those in the control group. As noted earlier, excessive rates of gallstones were also observed among participants in the clofibrate trial. Again the culprit is not clear. Was it the fats and the drug, or the lower cholesterol levels? Whichever the case, objective scientific evidence from numerous sources shows that lowering cholesterol carries important but poorly understood risk.

Finally, studies from Japan raise the question whether low cholesterol levels increase the risk of stroke. As much as the American researchers admired what seemed to be the effect of the Japanese diet in keeping serum cholesterol levels and heart disease deaths far below those found in the United States, other characteristics were not so desirable. Japan experienced far higher rates of stroke and cancer than the United States. Heart institute researchers apparently believed they could achieve one effect of imitating the Japanese diet without the others. But Japanese epidemiologists weren't so sure. In the journal *Preventive Medicine* they published a study that showed in rural communities where cholesterol levels were below 180 mg/dl, the rates of stroke were two to three times higher than areas with higher cholesterol levels. (The Japanese experts described the diets that produced typical serum cholesterol levels of 167 as "grossly inadequate.") Once again heart institute researchers pounced on this unwelcome news with a torrent of objection and cautions about leaping to conclusions. In fact, the evidence is far from conclusive, in part because so little is known about the low cholesterol levels the heart institute is aggressively pushing the American public to achieve.

Thus, a sea of uncertainty surrounds the territory of cholesterol levels below 200 mg/dl. Despite decades of clinical trials with a multitude of strategies, the sad fact remained that none of them had lowered cholesterol enough to provide an opportunity to understand either risks or benefits of low cholesterol levels. The trials selected only individuals with extremely high cholesterol levels, and failed to alter those levels by much. The most aggressive dieting lowered cholesterol only 5 to 7 percent. Drugs fared only modestly better: from 8 to 10 percent. So the frank fact remains that little is known about what happens after a dramatic lowering of cholesterol.

This might have remained a mostly hypothetical question had not the Food and Drug Administration approved in September 1987 a powerful new cholesterol-lowering drug called lovastatin. Merck Sharp & Dohme's new drug was apparently so much more effective than other approved drugs that in theory at least it might change the entire character of the cholesterol-lowering question. As one heart institute expert put it, lovastatin looked almost too good to be true. At a maximal dose it appeared to lower cholesterol by nearly one third, or at least twice as much as its competitors. Furthermore, because it was administered orally in two small pills, lovastatin had none of the adherence problems of cholestyramine which required patients to swallow millions of tiny indigestible plastic beads every day.

So here at last was a drug with the potential for resolving the cholesterol controversy in a decisive manner. It was just possible that cholesterol-level changes of this magnitude might at last provide the conclusive evidence of a capacity to save lives. If, on the other hand, experimenters had simply refused to face the lessons of more than twenty trials—that any substance powerful enough to lower cholesterol substantially also produces undesirable effects that outstrip the benefits—this theory also could also be put to the test.

It was thus unfortunate—and perhaps at great risk—that lovastatin was approved and is now rapidly spreading into widespread use without any information about its long-term effects, without any objective trials to measure its effect on heart disease, and without the systematic monitoring of side effects that occurs only in a large, long-term clinical trial. The heart institute drew up a plan to test lovastatin in the elderly, but at this writing has shelved the trial.

While the heart institute was not willing to test lovastatin it may have become the drug's most important but unwitting promoter. The National Cholesterol Education Program does not recommend lovastatin because of uncertainty about its long-term safety. But it is so difficult to persuade patients to take cholestyramine that the unintended effect will be to place millions of persons on long-term lovastatin therapy.

The experts who have evaluated this drug thus far have pronounced the known side effects acceptable in both number of people affected and severity. However, it is still worth examining the reasons why lovastatin deserves careful scrutiny.

Both the great appeal and potential hazard of lovastatin come from how it works. As was noted earlier, the liver is both the biggest consumer and manufacturer of cholesterol compounds in the human body. Lovastatin inhibits the liver's capacity to synthesize its own cholesterol. Therefore the liver must obtain its large cholesterol needs by absorbing greater quantities from the bloodstream; serum cholesterol levels plunge as a result.

Although lovastatin was heralded as a revolutionary new drug when approved in September 1987 such cholesterol synthesis inhibitors are not new, nor was previous experience encouraging. The first such drug was called triparanol, and it was voted the most important advance in clinical medicine in 1961. When some physicians, including the prominent Los Angeles cardiologist Eliot Corday, warned that it might be hazardous, they were studiously ignored by eager clinicians who embraced a new tool to lower cholesterol. Major authorities enthusiastically endorsed it. Two years later the drug was hastily withdrawn because of severe side effects, including rapid formation of cataracts, severe skin disorders, and heavy loss of hair. It might have become a celebrated public scandal rather than a minor historical note had not the news media's attention been so raptly focused on another drug just marketed by the same company. It was called thalidomide.

The second inhibitor was called compactin, and it appeared at almost the same time that lovastatin was first being tested in lipid laboratories. The earliest journal articles often mention them together. It was rapidly approved for use in Japan. And like triparanol it was hastily withdrawn. The reasons are not known. The sole clue to its ill effects comes from the heart institute's Basil M. Rifkind.

"It was hastily withdrawn, under a veil of secrecy," Rifkind told the institute's advisory council, "and no explicit statements have come out with respect to it. The problem there, however, appears to have surrounded some neoplasms [cancer] in dogs."

The possibility of still another association between cholesterol lowering and cancer might have raised questions when lovastatin came up for approval before an FDA advisory committee. However, the most serious new question raised at the committee review was whether lovastatin might cause heart attacks rather than prevent them. This characteristic had been previously observed in another cholesterol-lowering drug, dextrothyroxine, but was not discovered until the systematic monitoring that occurred in a heart institute clinical trial. In a letter to the committee considering lovastatin, member Saul Genuth said:

"The most important safety issue is that of the twelve cardiovascular deaths and twenty-four serious cardiovascular events recorded in approximately 1000 patients. The sponsor simply dismisses these as unrelated to drug administration."

Then, in one of those wry medical understatements, Genuth said, "If perchance, by some mechanism, the drug itself can cause myocardial infarction [heart attacks], then the benefit-to-risk ratio may be considerably lower than the sponsor projects in this application."

The advisory committee did not pursue the issue with Merck, perhaps because Genuth was not present to press the case, and Genuth did not oppose approval of the drug. It voted to approve lovastatin, intended for use over a lifetime even though the only long-term experience with the drug was limited to 200 persons who had taken the drug for a period of at least two years. The major clinical trial had lasted only twelve weeks. Lovastatin became the most rapidly approved drug in the FDA's history.

By mid-1988 Merck had concluded a trial comparing lovastatin to cholestyramine and published the result in the *Journal of the American Medical Association*. It concluded lovastatin was "both more effective and better tolerated" than cholestyramine.

The trial lasted only twelve weeks. In that brief time, among 176 patients taking lovastatin, there was one fatal heart attack, two non-fatal heart attacks, and one episode of severe chest pain requiring hospitalization. A single case of angina occurred among the patients taking cholestyramine. This trial is too short and has too few patients to pass normal statistical tests. But it is surprising that the authors did not comment.

Meanwhile, fragmentary data about the adverse effects of lovastatin continued to accumulate. If both animal and human experience is included, potential hazards of lovastatin include heart attacks, cancer, stroke, liver damage, cataracts, and severe muscle pain and damage. Just emerging in 1988 was new evidence of effects on the cholesterol-rich brain. The package insert warns that insomnia may be observed as an occasional side effect.

In a letter to the *New England Journal of Medicine* one physician noted a milder but much more frequent effect on the brain: "In our clinics we have observed no inability to sleep in patients taking lovastatin, but nine of fifty-one patients taking the drug (17.9 percent) have reported a shortening of their sleep period from one to three hours. It is known that lovastatin does cross the blood-brain barrier."

This account of the possible hazards of lovastatin was assembled from meeting transcripts, letters, and other materials not easily available to conscientious physicians. If they wanted to learn about the risks and benefits of lovastatin, they might have read the summary that appeared in the *New England Journal of Medicine*, written by Scott Grundy. In a laudatory nine-page article, Grundy devotes just five paragraphs to adverse effects, concluding that drugs that work like lovastatin "produce no important short-term side effects in most patients with hypercholesterolemia. . . ." He concludes, however, by saying that until more is known about the drug physicians should monitor their patients for evidence of damage to muscles and the liver.*

The problem is that the most important facts about lovastatin remain unknown. There are no immediate and tangible benefits from lowering cholesterol. No painful symptoms will disappear. No invading bacteria will be killed. If it has benefits, they will occur over the long term and be reflected in fewer heart attacks and fewer deaths. If there are serious dangers, such as heart attacks, cancer, or stroke, these too will be reflected only in the long term, and discovered only through the systematic study of a randomized trial lasting years. Voluntary reporting of side effects to the drug manufacturer or occasional letters in the medical journals are simply not systematic or thorough enough to provide conclusive evidence. Lovastatin could be a breakthrough drug. Or like so many previously tested cholesterol-lowering drugs, it could do more harm than good. The tragedy is we probably won't know. By late 1988, Merck reported at least 350,000 people were taking lovastatin, and it is reasonable to assume the number will climb daily. But it would be hard to find a case where so many Americans were going to be exposed to a powerful drug where nothing was known about either its long-term risks or its long-term benefits.

The biggest long-term cost of the National Cholesterol Education Program may be its delay of the search for a better understanding of heart disease. "We're near the pinnacle," cardiologist Eliot Corday had warned the heart institute. "Don't cast present concepts in concrete." But despite the deeply flawed evidence, the nation's most important medical authority and principal source of research grants had declared, in effect, the case was closed. The major cause of heart disease was elevated levels of serum cholesterol, specifically LDL. The ink was barely dry on that declaration when the truth of Corday's prophetic warning became apparent.

From Helsinki, Finland, came a clinical trial that was the most successful yet in reducing coronary heart disease. Here was an experiment that on its face finally met the standards for the long-sought golden fleece

---

*Unlike the heart, the liver has a substantial capacity to replace damaged or destroyed tissue.

of heart research: a 30 percent reduction in coronary heart disease that also met the usual statistical tests. Like the other trials it had no effect on total mortality or life expectancy, but the Helsinki trial was the most promising effort yet. It used a drug called gemfibrozil, a chemical relative of clofibrate, and was conducted among Finnish men with severely elevated cholesterol. Although the Helsinki trial was a success in the battle to prevent coronary heart disease, it was also a distinct setback for the heart institute's official view that LDL was the culprit. The most powerful effect of gemfibrozil was to raise levels of high density lipoproteins, or HDL, the so-called good cholesterol.

Other evidence also supported the importance of HDL. Studies of the positive effects of exercise showed the key benefit was probably raising HDL levels. Coronary heart disease begins to develop in young men at puberty primarily because of a sharp drop in HDL levels not experienced by women. The Framingham researchers had found that low HDL was a more accurate predictor of coronary heart disease than high levels of other cholesterol compounds, especially LDL. Even though gemfibrozil was apparently twice as effective as cholestyramine in reducing coronary heart disease, this didn't affect the heart institute's position. Basil Rifkind, writing in the *New England Journal of Medicine,* appeared uncomfortable because gemfibrozil didn't reduce LDL. He said, "It is difficult at present to define its precise place in the treatment scheme because of its variable effect on levels of LDL cholesterol." He urged the nation's physicians to continue to follow the heart institute's guidelines or in effect to ignore the trial. Gemfibrozil fared little better at the FDA, where an expert committee concluded its benefits in preventing heart disease did not outweigh its risks. Despite these setbacks in the health establishment, HDL remains a promising new frontier. But whether the issue is further trials of the powerful new lovastatin or accelerated research into HDL, progress towards better prevention of heart disease cannot help but be slowed by those who have erroneously convinced themselves they already know the answer.

•••

FEAR OF DYING is the lever that will be used to move millions into treatment for high cholesterol. The descriptive terms are simultaneously frightening and vague. "You are at high risk of dying of a heart attack." "You have dangerously high cholesterol." When backed by health authorities and aggressively promoted to the public these are frightening words indeed. Thus the final perspective on cholesterol is the simplest one: What is the actual impact on life expectancy of high or low cholesterol? How great a danger to life do we face? Surprising answers to this question emerge from the same body of heart institute research that forms the scientific basis of much of what is known about cholesterol.

While the elaborate and lengthy MR.FIT trial failed to demonstrate benefits of strict dieting, quitting smoking, or lower blood pressure in preventing heart attack deaths, a spin-off project was to have great influence. To select the highest risk subjects for MR.FIT, the investigators had to screen 361,662 middle-aged men as possible candidates. A team led by Jeremiah Stamler of Northwestern University continued to follow this entire group and calculate death rates and survival. While it relied on frequently unreliable death certificates and a single cholesterol measurement, its size alone was impressive. It was seventy times larger than the Framingham study, twenty years more recent, and included participants from eighteen cities rather than a single Massachusetts town. The MR.FIT spin-off spawned one of the most frequently repeated slogans of the cholesterol reduction campaigners: Each 1 percent reduction in cholesterol will lead to a 2 percent reduction in the risk of dying of coronary heart disease.* The researchers also found no particular threshold where the danger leaped higher, just a steady increase in the risk of heart disease as cholesterol levels rose. Furthermore, one fifth of the men with the highest cholesterol levels were about three times more likely to die of heart disease than a similar number with the lowest cholesterol levels. The study has since become an important empirical building block of the assault on cholesterol.

• • •

---

*The actual finding was technically the reverse: that for each 1 percent increase in cholesterol level, the risk of coronary heart disease increased 2 percent.

It was thus surprising that a major scientific research article, published in an important journal, the *Journal of the American Medical Association,* contained such a significant omission. To many, the critical question is how does high cholesterol or low cholesterol affect life expectancy? In short, what was the total mortality? The answer to this question can be deduced from a later report from the group.

This is what the complete data show, calculated from a table published the next year:

Serum Cholesterol	Alive	All Deaths	CHD Deaths
		Percent	
Low (202 mg/dl or less)	97.8	2.2	0.5
Average (203 to 244 mg/dl)	97.3	2.7	0.9
High (245 mg/dl or more)	96.2	3.8	1.7

(361,662 men followed for 7 years)

When examining total mortality, and not just deaths from coronary heart disease, the hazards of high cholesterol appear considerably more modest. Further, these figures apply to only a minority of those at risk: young and middle-aged men. As noted earlier, the relationship is weak or non-existent among the elderly, where most heart disease deaths occur, and among pre-menopausal women, where the disease is rare.

A team of physicians and researchers at Harvard University used the MR.FIT and Framingham data to answer the broad question of the benefits of lowering cholesterol through diet. Using the risk factor equations from Framingham and the diet results of the MR.FIT trial, the researchers calculated the benefits of a lifelong program of cholesterol dieting. The team, led by William C. Taylor, published the results in the *Annals of Internal Medicine.* For persons without other risk factors, such as smoking or high blood pressure, they concluded:

"We calculate a gain in life expectancy of from three days to three months from a lifelong program of cholesterol reduction."

Taylor and his coauthors also expressed concern that they might be overstating the benefits of cholesterol reduction because they assumed that any reduction in the risk of heart disease would not be offset by other increased risk.

In an accompanying editorial, Marshall Becker of the University of Michigan said: "We should make more effective and efficient use of our resources and regain public confidence by concentrating on a few areas in which deleterious effects on health are clear and profound, such as smoking prevention and cessation, alcohol and drug abuse, and gross obesity."

The widely discussed article triggered the inevitable rebuttal from the heart institute. However, Taylor's defense was persuasive: He noted that heart institute researchers in Framingham had just published an analysis of cholesterol and life expectancy that was even more pessimistic than his own. That study was equally revealing.

Four decades after the Framingham study began, the research team examined the question of total mortality and cholesterol. The results once again showed that death from other causes mostly offset any risks of high cholesterol. Among men, after age forty-seven, the researchers found "there is no increase in overall mortality with either high or low cholesterol." Among women there was no relationship, except among those aged forty to forty-seven when the trial began. Furthermore, the researchers revealed that people whose cholesterol levels are declining may be at special risk. "After age fifty years the association of mortality with cholesterol values is confounded by people whose cholesterol levels are falling—perhaps due to diseases predisposing to death." Left unanswered was how a spontaneous decline "might" predispose one to death, but a non-spontaneous response to treatment would not.

Marshall Becker summed up succinctly the implications that neither the clinical trials nor the epidemiological studies suggested a relationship between cholesterol and life expectancy.

"The effect of all our interventions may be analogous to stewards rearranging the deck chairs on the *Titanic*," he said.

Finally, what was the likely role of cholesterol in the phenomenal rise and decline in coronary heart disease? From World War II until 1963 the mortality rate from coronary heart disease rose steadily and alarmingly. Then it declined steeply throughout the 1970s and into early 1980s. By 1986, the death rate was 42 percent lower than the 1963 peak. The causes of these enormous changes have never been convincingly explained. But one factor can be ruled out: cholesterol. From 1960 to 1980, there was virtually no change in the average serum cholesterol levels in the American population. Over twenty years cholesterol levels declined very slightly, leaving the average in 1980 just 3 percent lower than 1960. Thus cholesterol levels remained virtually unchanged during a twenty-year period in which deaths from heart disease first rose and then declined dramatically. Whatever had saved so many thousands of lives, it was clear that cholesterol could not be included as an important contributor.

TREATMENT

7
A LOT CAN
GO WRONG

Aaron Yochelson's heart is about to stop beating.

At the moment, it is pulsing sixty-two times a minute in his exposed chest cavity, the bright yellow fat deposits on its surface gleaming under the operating room lights at the Washington Hospital Center.

Heart surgeon Jorge M. Garcia closes a stainless steel clamp over the aorta, the main artery that carries blood from the heart to the rest of the body. Next he is handed a short needle attached to a long flexible tube leading to a plastic bag filled with deadly poison—chilled potassium chloride and water. He plunges the needle in, and the fluid pours into the heart. Immediately it begins to beat more feebly. Garcia pours a bag of almost frozen salt water over the outside of the heart muscle. It sloshes around in the sack of white tissue that surrounds the heart. The muscle twitches a few more times and is still.

Yochelson is surrounded by eight specialists who are about to perform the first of that day's six coronary artery bypass operations. For the actual cutting, Garcia works with two assistants who are not physicians but who perform surgical work under his direction. The team is rounded out by the anesthesiologist and an assistant, the operator of the heart/lung pump, and two nurses.

In this room crowded with bright lights, medical hardware, and people, Yochelson has become invisible as a real person. The transformation was quick and efficient. Minutes earlier, he was a pleasant, balding seventy-year-old man in a white hospital gown. As soon as he was unconscious the two nurses took over. He was stripped naked, and his body scrubbed from head to toe with purple cleaning solution. Catheters and other tubes were quickly inserted into practically every natural entrance or exit of the body, and into several new openings created for this operation. Then Yochelson began to disappear. His head was hidden when a stainless steel instrument stand was placed over his head and draped with sterile blue surgical cloths. Soon blue cloths cloaked the rest of his body, leaving just two areas exposed—the chest, and an area of his upper thigh. Even these are covered with a thin translucent plastic film, leaving nothing in view that looks like a living person.

Now, with a murmur of satisfaction, Garcia reaches into Yochelson's chest cavity and gently holds the limp heart in his hand and examines it. "See, it has relaxed," he says.

Minutes before Garcia sawed open Yochelson's chest he had carefully reviewed reruns of X-ray movies of Yochelson's heart, taken three weeks earlier. As the arteries pulsated with each beat of the heart, the film showed blockages in three places: in the main artery on the right side of the heart, in the longest branch off the left main coronary artery, and in the vessel that loops around the heart from front to back.

Yochelson will get three bypass grafts.

While Garcia opened the chest, Jimmy Weigler, a surgical assistant, cut open Yochelson's right leg, from groin to knee, to harvest segments of vein to be used in the bypass.

Just as Garcia gets the heart stopped, Weigler has a six-inch piece of vein ready. He has clamped one end shut and used a syringe to fill it with fluid, to check for leaks and preserve the tissue.

Now begins the part of the operation where the surgeon's skill can make the difference between life and death. Garcia will splice the end of the vein onto the artery on Yochelson's heart. The artery runs down the surface of the heart muscle on the right side. It is less than one tenth of an inch in diameter on the inside, hard to see and now collapsed flat on the surface of the heart muscle because no blood flows through it. Garcia uses a curved surgical needle less than a half inch long. Far too small to be held, the needle is inserted in a holder that Garcia grips with a long gold-handled forceps.

Garcia cannot do this alone. Across from him is his first surgical assistant, Bob Gilbert, who has joined him in more than 3,000 heart operations. Their four hands move as if driven by a common mind. Gilbert holds, Garcia stitches. Garcia stitches, Gilbert ties. It takes twelve tiny stitches to form a "T" junction between the vein and the artery.

If his stitch is a millimeter too deep, Garcia could sew the artery shut, cutting off almost half the blood supply to the heart.

When he has finished it looks as if the end of a piece of red spaghetti has been sewn onto the surface of Yochelson's heart.

It has taken twelve minutes of non-stop work. Speed is important. The heart muscle is getting no blood, no oxygen. While cooled and bathed in salt water to minimize damage, the tissue is in danger of slowly beginning to die.

The next two grafts go somewhat faster. The last one, however, looks particularly difficult. Gilbert has to lift the heart so Garcia can graft the third piece of vein in place on the back side of the heart.

As he nears the end of the most demanding part of the surgery, Garcia relieves the tension with surgeon's humor.

"Back in the early days of bypass surgery, the surgeon would yell at the assistant if he dropped the heart," he says.

It is not hard to see what he means. If the slippery mass of heart should slide out of Gilbert's hands, back into the chest cavity, the careful stitching would be ruined and Garcia would have to start over.

Weigler, who is starting to sew up Yochelson's right leg, says, "You never dropped the heart, did you?"

"Certainly I would never admit it," says Garcia.

During the operation the natural functions of Yochelson's body have been suppressed. He is unconscious. Every muscle in his body except the heart has been paralyzed with a drug that works like curare. The heartbeat was suppressed with potassium chloride. His body temperature has been lowered to 86°F, which under other circumstances would soon kill him. To turn over all the vital body functions to the array of machines that surround him it was first necessary to disable all his own natural equipment.

The return flow of blood is still being collected as usual, in the right atrium of his heart. From there it flows into a length of clear plastic tubing that leads to the mechanical heart/lung machine, located directly behind Garcia. The pumping is accomplished in a hollow cylinder lined with a spiral coil of flexible plastic tubing. A rotating paddle gently squeezes the blood forward, into a reservoir where it is oxygenated and, right now, cooled. Another tube leads back to Yochelson and flows into the aorta on the other side of the clamp that Garcia squeezed closed at the beginning of the operation.

A tiny malfunction in this equipment can quickly kill or injure. During a similar operation at Methodist Hospital in Indianapolis somehow the blood level in the reservoir fell too low for just a second. An air bubble entered the bloodstream and went to the brain, leaving the patient permanently in a "chronic vegetative state."

After testing each graft for leaks, Garcia releases the clamp over the aorta, and blood supplied by the mechanical pump flows into the heart. Exactly twenty-six minutes after it stopped, Yochelson's heart begins to beat feebly again.

But they are far from done. The heart is not yet pumping blood. The grafts are attached only to the surface arteries, and the other ends, pinched off with white plastic clamps, dangle in the chest cavity.

Garcia begins to attach the loose ends of the grafts to the aorta, now secured partly closed by a clamp that permits some blood to nourish the heart. He already has punched one hole in the aorta when he first injected the potassium fluid to stop the heart. Now he punches two more holes in a neat row ending less than an inch from the heart.

As he stitches the grafts in place Garcia also sews around each a stainless steel ring to mark the location of the new arteries. Should Yochelson have more heart trouble—a common occurrence—the rings will identify the grafts so the blood flow through the new plumbing can be monitored.

Now, his stitching complete, Garcia bleeds the air out of the grafts with a needle to get them ready to deliver blood to the heart muscle. Letting a tiny bubble of air into the bloodstream can cause a fatal stroke if the air bubble reaches the brain. He has arrived at the pivotal moment most likely to determine whether Yochelson will live or die.

The point of highest risk comes when the heart is asked to begin delivering blood to the body again. Invariably, open-heart surgery must damage a muscle that was already weakened by disease. If the operation has fatally damaged the heart, rather than repairing it, now is when the team is most likely to find out.

Two key members of the surgical team have been silently preparing for this moment. Angie Nevaldine is the perfusionist who runs the mechanical heart/lung pump. Dongzin Hur is the anesthesiologist, who must manage a constantly changing mixture of drugs that control or suppress breathing, thin or thicken the blood, and manage the level of unconsciousness.

"Ready to go off bypass?" asks Garcia, looking at Hur and Nevaldine.

Hur is not ready. He wants to give Yochelson another minute on a slightly different mix of drugs.

The minute passes. "How's your temperature?" Garcia asks Nevaldine. She nods. To minimize damage, body temperature was earlier lowered by cooling the blood flowing through the pump. But it must be returned nearly to normal to help the heart resume its function.

"OK," says Garcia, and slowly Yochelson's heart is returned to service. Nevaldine, operating the controls of the pump, gradually lets Yochelson's heart take over. It has been just fifty-seven minutes since his heart stopped.

All eyes now are on the monitors showing Yochelson's heart functions in five rows of blips marching across the screens. The third row is the critical one, measuring not only the heartbeat, but the volume of blood being pumped. That row of blips will indicate whether Yochelson's heart can still pump enough blood to sustain his life.

Slowly the spikes begin to appear on the monitor, and soon all five indicators show the heart to be functioning as it pulses powerfully in the exposed chest cavity. Yochelson has started on his way to recovery.

Quickly Garcia disconnects the mechanical pump. He sloshes a beaker of warm salt water over the heart and Gilbert suctions it off. He installs wiring for a pacemaker, in case the heartbeat should become erratic. With a short piece of plastic tube he creates a drain for any post-operative bleeding in the chest cavity. Now the team starts down the home stretch, closing up Yochelson's chest.

"See? Cheap equipment! A shoemaker's awl and a kitchen spoon," says Garcia as he holds up the tools he will use to close the chest.

On one side Gilbert punches a hole through the breastbone with the shoemaker's awl while Garcia holds a kitchen spoon under it so the awl won't puncture the heart or an artery. Then a length of twenty-gauge stainless steel wire is drawn back through the hole. They reverse roles on the other side of the chest, and then Gilbert twists the wires together and tightens them with pliers.

William J. Fouty, chief of surgery, strolls into the operating room to check up on things.

He kids Garcia. "This still the same patient?" While accuracy is paramount, surgeons pride themselves on their dexterity and speed, and this operation has taken sixty-seven minutes, slightly longer than average for Garcia.

Fouty points at Yochelson, who is going to wake up soon.

"You know, so far he hasn't felt a thing. But when he wakes up he is *not* going to feel good. I can tell you that."

Fouty, veteran of thousands of operations, is remembering the similar bypass operation that was performed on him. And he winces.

• • •

FUTURE HISTORIANS MAY fault late twentieth-century America not for its failings, but for the casual manner in which it took extraordinary achievements for granted. Aaron Yochelson's remarkable operation, and the thousands like it performed every month, deserve a prominent position in the catalogue of major achievements not only of medicine, but of our whole society. A brief look at other pages in the catalogue of unappreciated wonders may help focus on why open-heart surgery deserves to be ranked so high.

The first person in the front row of a modern symphony orchestra holds a wooden box capable of emitting a sound of subtlety and beauty, but only because of a lifetime of daily dedication. The pitch must be played to tolerances of 1/400th, and every note must be timed correctly to a fraction of a second. In a symphony, he must produce about 9,000 such notes without a mistake. He will be joined by one hundred others facing acoustical and coordination demands of similar magnitude. Since childhood each player has demonstrated unusual talent mixed with uncommon dedication. These virtuoso individual performances must merge flawlessly into a seamless whole. For an example of skill, coordination, and teamwork, it would be hard to surpass this feat. It would also be difficult to find another that has changed less in the last two hundred years.

To focus on technological achievements alone might lead us to giant supercomputers, electron microscopes, or orbiting communications satellites. While wondrous are these machines, we are careful not to trust them too much. We expect large computers to break down, and are not surprised when spacecraft fail. Computer error is a more familiar part of the modern vocabulary than computer achievement.

To observe technology and teamwork unified in an unforgiving environment, drive to the end of the runway at a metropolitan airport. Watch an endless sequence of 150-ton vehicles, hurtling through three dimensional space, drop gracefully on a small patch of concrete at sixty-eight-second intervals. However, this impressive achievement is mostly a demonstration of the modern ability to divide a complex process into simpler tasks that can be mastered by a team of average persons with modest training. This is no job for amateurs, but professional flight trainers insist they can train almost anyone to land a commercial aircraft.

But not just anyone can be a heart surgeon. The task requires a particular blend of forceful personality, manual dexterity, and mental discipline; and this effort must be flawlessly blended with the efforts of the entire surgical team. With a human life invariably at stake, bypass surgery may be the most unforgiving environment of all. To dare to make extensive modifications of such a critical organ requires supreme confidence matched by mastery over many of the vital processes of life. And this achievement is not a one-time spectacular, a Notre Dame cathedral of medicine, but a standard service routinely available in every community of even modest size. In heart surgery is the rosy image of medicine as it would like to see itself.

That same great achievement also reflects many of the stark failings of American medicine. To understand those failings, and see why they coexist with such excellence requires a deeper look at bypass surgery, the medical problem it was developed to solve, and what is known about its major limitations.

• • •

TWO CENTURIES BEFORE physicians dreamed of bypass surgery they first identified a disease that was characterized by periodic chest pains. The ailment has an official medical name, angina pectoris, which means strangling in the chest, and it afflicts three million Americans. As the network of coronary arteries becomes obstructed by buildups of fat, fiber, and calcium, portions of the heart muscle can become oxygen-starved, particularly when the body demands a greater output from the heart pump. Some individuals experience pain under these circumstances, and the symptoms range from a mild tightness in the chest to excruciating and debilitating pain. Initially these pains occur at intervals, often after exercise, eating, excitement, or stress. As the obstructions increase in size over time the pains may become more severe and frequent and may occur without any triggering event. Sufferers from angina are at increased risk from two life-threatening events: the disruption of the heart's electrical rhythm that leads to sudden cardiac death, and formation of a clot that abruptly and completely blocks an artery, destroying part of the heart muscle.

The first challenge that angina posed to physicians was correctly identifying the disease. Persons with extensive lesions in their coronary artery do not necessarily suffer from angina. For many the first warning symptom of coronary heart disease is a heart attack. Why an insufficient supply of blood produces sharp pains in some individuals and no symptoms in others remains a major unsolved mystery. As a final confounding factor, chest pains are symptoms commonly reported by persons who have nothing wrong with their heart whatsoever. For the unwary physician angina can be easily confused with anxiety, hyperventilation, heartburn, ulcers, and inflammation of the gallbladder. When experts at twelve medical schools directly examined the coronary arteries of a large group of patients under treatment for angina, they discovered that 28 percent did not have coronary heart disease. The diagnosis had been in error. The most pressing problem of many years' standing, however, was not the ambiguity of the symptoms but the urgent need for an effective treatment.

For many decades nitroglycerine was the principal—and perhaps only—useful treatment for angina pectoris. A tablet, dissolved under the tongue, usually relieved the angina pains in one to two minutes. So close was the relationship that some medical texts define angina pectoris as those chest pains that disappear quickly with nitroglycerine. But while it relieves symptoms, it has no long term effect on the underlying condition, which in a distressingly large number of patients grows steadily worse. And so it was that doctors turned to surgeons for a solution, for something that would more permanently relieve the angina pains.

The early surgical attempts to cure angina can be fairly described as somewhere between crude and ludicrous. In 1922 a French surgeon tried severing the nerve that carried the pain signals. Not surprisingly, it eliminated the pain but had no effect on the underlying condition. A decade later a team of four surgeons reported that removing the thyroid, eliminating the stimulation of its powerful hormones, limited sudden demands on the heart. It too reduced angina pains, but the patients soon suffered symptoms of thyroid deficiency. Shortly after World War II other surgical approaches were proposed that made slightly more physiological and anatomical sense. An operation that attracted worldwide attention involved two blood vessels quite close to the heart that are embedded in the chest wall. They are called the internal mammary arteries.

While the internal mammaries do not directly supply the heart with blood, some surgeons believed that tiny branches off the mammaries might interconnect with branches of the coronary arteries, creating what is called collateral circulation. The objective of the operation was to create—or increase—that collateral circulation. Through incisions between the second and third ribs it was possible to reach the two arteries and tie a suture tightly around them. The idea was, by choking off the downstream flow, to force all the blood entering these arteries down the tiny branches nearest the heart and then into the coronary arteries. It had additional appeal from a technical standpoint because it was not necessary to open the chest and enter the thoracic cavity. This was a simple operation that could be quickly learned by almost any general surgeon. The procedure was called ligation (or tying off) of the internal mammary arteries, and pioneering surgeons who tried it were soon reporting dramatic results in research articles published in major medical journals in the late 1950s.

For example, in the *American Journal of Cardiology*, J. R. Kitchell reported that 36 percent of 135 ligation patients experienced complete relief of angina. In *Northwest Medicine*, I. C. Brill found that eleven out of eighteen patients reported complete disappearance of symptoms. Others followed with their own research, and soon the popular press joined the growing wave of enthusiasm for the new treatment. *Reader's Digest* featured an article, "New Surgery for Ailing Hearts."

However, Leonard A. Cobb, a young Seattle cardiologist, was more skeptical. It wasn't clear to him why the operation relieved angina pains. Nor was it clear whether collateral circulation was in fact taking place. It does occur between the coronary arteries that supply the heart muscle, but it was not anatomically clear that such a structure existed between the coronary arteries and the internal mammaries. Working with four other physicians at the University of Washington, Cobb devised an experiment.

Cobb found seventeen patients with angina who agreed to participate in the study of a new treatment whose value, they were told, was uncertain. (An investigator's enthusiasm for a new therapy may be sufficient to help some patients improve, regardless of the effects of the treatment itself.)

Each of the seventeen patients was wheeled into the operating room under local anesthesia. Before he began to work the surgeon was handed an envelope with a card giving him instructions. The surgeon performed the complete operation for eight of the patients. In nine cases the surgeon appeared to proceed as usual. The incisions were made. The mammary arteries were isolated. But in these cases the arteries were not actually tied off. It was a sham operation. The physicians who would monitor the progress of the seventeen patients did not know which patient was which. All the patients believed they had received the complete operation.

Next Cobb and his colleagues sought to measure the progress of the patients more scientifically and objectively than in previous studies. Some dramatic improvement occurred, just as earlier researchers had reported. In one group the patients reported needing to take 43 percent fewer nitroglycerine tablets to relieve chest pains. On the average their tolerance for exercise improved in carefully monitored tests. One patient showed a particularly dramatic change. His angina pains disappeared entirely. Before the operation his electrocardiogram showed abnormalities after only four minutes of exercise—key evidence that the heart was not getting enough oxygen. Afterward his ECG was normal. Another patient, previously so wracked by chest pains that he couldn't work, returned to his former occupation. However, not a single one of these patients actually received the complete operation.

The patients who did get the full operation reported roughly equivalent improvement. If for one half the subjects the operation was literally a sham, why did all the patients feel better?

In all the studies the patients experienced improvement in the critical but subjective *symptom* of angina. And they took only about half as many nitroglycerine tablets for pain relief. For some patients there was objective evidence that the operation worked—changes in the electrocardiogram attesting to an actual reduction in the oxygen starvation of the heart after exercise. This is the placebo effect of surgery. Henry K. Beecher of the Harvard Medical School explained why this happens.

"The situation prevailing before, during, and after surgery is one usually filled with grave anxiety and stress. It would be surprising if, in this charged atmosphere, surgery did not have a powerful placebo action, in addition to what it may or may not accomplish physiologically."

This devastating clinical trial caused the internal mammary ligation to fade quickly from the scene, but the flow of more draconian but dubious surgical treatments continued.

One of the most impressive results in the relief of angina came from a surgical procedure in which the outer layer of the heart muscle was removed. Then the exposed muscle was abraded with asbestos until it was bloody. As the deliberately damaged heart healed up again, according to the theory, the muscle would obtain additional supplies of blood from the vessels embedded in the fibrous sack that surrounds it. In 1958 Claude S. Beck reported in the *Journal of the American Medical Association* that 97 percent of the patients upon whom he had operated experienced relief of angina pains.

A surgical approach that sounds even more bizarre than Beck's enjoyed much greater popularity. It was called the internal mammary implant, and was enthusiastically promoted by its inventor, a Canadian heart surgeon named Arthur M. Vineberg. Like others before him, Vineberg turned to the internal mammary arteries lying so temptingly close to the heart. But Vineberg didn't intend to depend on the chance that a small collateral flow of blood might exist between the mammaries and the coronary arteries. He was going to fashion a direct connection. In the Vineberg procedure a tunnel was carved through the heart muscle and the internal mammary artery was then pushed into the tunnel and sutured into place. The idea was that, like a sapling plunged into fertile soil, the mammary would sprout connections with tiny branches of the coronary arteries.

Vineberg relentlessly promoted the remarkable changes that occurred in his patients: "An oil prospector . . . could walk through the bush for miles with a packsack after the operation. A Grey Nun nursing sister who, two years prior to the operation was totally disabled by angina . . . is now pain free and working a full day. A patient who is four years postoperative now ploughs 1,600 acres."

Few disbelieved the remarkable changes in angina symptoms achieved among Vineberg's patients. But many were skeptical that the internal mammary implant did much to increase the blood supply to the heart. Surgeons at Johns Hopkins performed the operation on twenty-five pigs and nineteen dogs. A viable junction between the mammary artery and the heart was found in only one pig and one dog. Forcing the heart to rely on blood flowing through the mammary artery quickly killed the others. As the procedure grew in popularity and underwent refinement more evidence emerged that on occasion, at least, the internal mammary implant could indeed supply substantial amounts of blood to the heart.

But did it prevent heart attacks? Would it prolong life? These were hardly trivial questions because the internal mammary procedure caused substantial loss of life. Vineberg reported operative deaths of 5.8 percent of his patients whose periodic chest pains were not increasing in frequency or severity. It is revealing that by 1972 the Vineberg operation had been in increasing use for twenty-seven years without an objective scientific test to determine whether it actually dealt with the underlying problem of coronary heart disease.

In 1972 academic researchers working with the Veterans Administration hospitals decided it was high time to try to answer the key question of whether either the Vineberg or Beck procedure improved the supply of blood to the heart sufficiently to prolong life. Then, at the last minute, they changed their minds. A new heart operation was growing like wildfire, and even less was known about the results *it* might achieve. So the researchers decided to focus on the hot new procedure. It was coronary artery bypass surgery.

From the time it was perfected in the late 1960s coronary bypass surgery was something of a dream come true. The surgical procedures that preceded bypass surgery were crude and clumsy not because of lack of imagination but because of severe limitations of technology. The early operations such as the Beck procedure had to be performed on a heart that was still beating, or completed in the few minutes that the patient could survive without a heartbeat. The heart/lung machine, which became widely available in the early 1960s, opened a whole new world of possibilities for delicate operations on the heart. The heart valves could now be replaced. Congenital defects could be repaired. But initially there still wasn't much that could be done for obstructions in the coronary arteries. It might be technically possible to bypass the obstructions, but the heart surgeons just couldn't find the blockages. They were hidden in the tiny and hard-to-reach coronary arteries that were collapsed flat while the patient was on the bypass machine. Then, at the Cleveland Clinic, F. Mason Sones put the last missing piece of the puzzle into place.

Sones was trying to figure out how to see into the coronary arteries. It was already possible to observe the valves and pumping chambers in operation. This was accomplished by inserting a long hollow tube through an artery in the arm and gently pushing it all the way into the left ventricle. Then a special dye was injected through the tube to make the pumping chamber visible on a fluoroscope screen. But he still couldn't see much of the tiny coronary arteries. Sones thought the answer might be a more powerful amplifier to produce a better image of the heart. But the device was so large and clumsy that he had to crawl into a hole beneath the patient to see the screen. One day he suddenly observed the right coronary artery standing out in such bright contrast he immediately realized a horrible mistake had been made.

His associate had accidentally lodged the end of the hollow tube directly in the narrow entrance to the artery, and injected a large quantity of the contrast medium.

"Pull it out," Sones called to his associate, and grabbed a scalpel. The enormous quantity of contrast medium, intended to fill a whole pumping chamber and then be quickly pumped away, would be so toxic to the heart muscle that he expected the heartbeat to halt completely. And within seconds it did.

Before taking the drastic step of opening the patient's chest to massage his heart, Sones tried something simpler. He told the still-conscious patient to cough. Sometimes the movement of the diaphragm will massage the heart enough that a normal heartbeat will resume. And in this case it did. So not only did Sones' patient survive, but also after using much smaller amounts of the special dye, he had learned how to see into the coronary arteries. A few years after Sones perfected the technique, a colleague at the Cleveland Clinic, Rene Favaloro, performed the first modern bypass operation. The year was 1968.

Bypass was quite different from the operations that preceded it. There was no more waiting for blood vessels to sprout mysterious connections. No more carving tunnels in the heart muscle for the internal mammary. This was plumbing, straight and simple. Segments of vein or artery would be stitched directly in place to bypass the obstruction and bring additional blood into the coronary arteries. With angiography the doubters could watch, and even measure, the additional flow of blood. It looked as if the problem of angina, waiting two hundred years for a viable solution, had an effective treatment at last.

All the elements were present for an explosion in open heart surgery. Here was a new treatment for a severe problem affecting millions of persons. Fueled by demand for valve replacement and repair of birth defects, heart surgery had already expanded. That meant a growing number of heart surgeons in training, pleased to embrace an operation for which demand might be almost unlimited. Thus starting in 1970 the volume of bypass surgery began to double every two years. By 1975 the number of operations performed each year had grown to 60,000. And by 1987 there were more than 230,000 bypass procedures annually, making it one of the most commonly performed major operations, at an annual cost of over five billion dollars.

In the meantime it was clear to cardiologists and surgeons that the bypass operation was dramatically effective in relieving angina pains. But when progress comes in medicine, memories often grow short about earlier techniques discredited or rapidly abandoned. So, little was heard about the fact that internal mammary ligation relieved angina, even when the operation was not actually performed. Nor was there much discussion about the Beck procedure of bloodying up the heart, and its 97 percent effectiveness. And Arthur Vineberg and other adherents of his procedure could still tout dozens of success stories about disabled patients who were now ploughing fields and hiking the wilds. In the bypass operation medicine seemed to have the answer at last, and heart surgeons were not reluctant to test that proposition in a randomized clinical trial. With a technique that observably increased the supply of blood to the heart through the same arteries that had been blocked, who could doubt that it would prevent heart attacks and prolong life? Numerous surgical procedures are in common use today whose benefits have never been objectively measured in a clinical trial. Bypass surgery was something of the exception, the new glamour treatment so promising but so expensive that it was well worth measuring the benefits precisely in terms of lives saved.

That's why there was such shock when the medical world opened the pages of the nation's most prestigious medical publication, the *New England Journal of Medicine,* in September of 1977. It described a devastatingly simple experiment. At thirteen Veterans Administration hospitals a total of 596 patients were identified for the study. Ninety-four percent had moderate or severe angina and two thirds had already suffered at least one severe heart attack. These were individuals with serious symptoms and advanced coronary heart disease. The patients were randomly divided into two groups. One was sent to bypass surgery. The other group was managed medically with nitroglycerine tablets and other drug therapy. At the end of three years the two groups were compared. Among those managed medically 87 percent were still alive. Among those treated surgically 86 percent were still living. The most important benefits of the dream treatment could not be demonstrated in an objective scientific experiment. Bypass surgery was not achieving its most important purpose, extending human life. That occurred in part because the benefits of the operation were offset by the 5.6 percent mortality rate from the surgery itself.

That was only the first of two surprises. The second was that this seminal revelation did not slow the rapid growth of bypass surgery for ever-larger numbers of patients with an even wider variety of conditions. To understand the reasons for the second surprise requires a look at the chaotic and uncontrolled process by which American medicine adopts innovations in treatment. This is most graphically illustrated by examining the important exception to customary medical practice, the testing and approval of new drugs.

If the new treatment happens to be a pharmacological substance, it must run a gauntlet of specifically prescribed testing before it can be offered for general use. In the first round of experiments, called Phase I testing, the new drug must be tested for safety, and the appropriate doses established. In Phase II the experimenter must demonstrate in further trials that the drug is reasonably effective. Finally, in Phase III, come randomized clinical trials. Like Cobb's experiment with internal mammary ligation, the trials are normally double-blind, meaning neither patient nor experimenter knows who receives the real drug and who gets a placebo. The involvement of several medical centers, as in the Veterans trial, protects against conscious or unconscious bias or outright cheating. Not only are three rounds of trials required, the entire process is regulated by a single agency, the federal Food and Drug Administration, which is advised by special panels of experts. This centralization means that a drug is either approved or it is not. If unexpected side effects occur or new evidence emerges, it does not become an interesting and controversial article in a medical journal— the drug is withdrawn from use. This process has critics who say it is unacceptably slow and delays the flow of valuable new treatments to the public. It also has opponents who believe it is too lax, that long-term effects aren't adequately studied, and the reporting of adverse effects is wholly inadequate. Perhaps drug approval is not a perfect system, but it is reasonable, open, consistent, and centralized.

None of this orderly testing process, which applies to drugs ranging from life-saving vaccines to acne ointment, had occurred with the introduction of a hazardous surgical treatment that immediately killed about one out of twenty patients. Individual physicians decide independently when to introduce or adopt a new procedure, and on whom to perform it. They may report their results in medical journals—or they may not. Some hospitals monitor such new procedures; others do not. If published research challenges the efficacy of a treatment, each individual physician interprets the results, deciding whether any change in his existing practice is necessary. When the results of the Veterans Administration trial appeared, each cardiologist and heart surgeon was left to decide what it meant for his practice, if anything. And while a simple operation like internal mammary ligation might be rapidly abandoned it was not clear this would happen with a procedure upon which so many livelihoods depended.

"This rapidly growing enterprise is developing a momentum and constituency of its own, and as time passes, it will be progressively more difficult to curtail it materially . . . ," wrote Harvard's Eugene Braunwald, a major authority in cardiology, in response to the Veterans trial.

There was also no central body, like the FDA, where the benefits and risks of a surgical procedure were systematically evaluated. It was literally every man for himself. The practice of introducing a treatment first and testing it later also transformed the character and atmosphere of the ensuing debate about bypass surgery.

Could a cardiologist who had personally recommended bypass surgery to hundreds of patients be objective in assessing the Veterans Administration clinical trial? And what kind of dispassionate judgment could reasonably be expected from the hundreds of heart surgeons who performed the operation, and had built professional reputations and personal livelihoods on bypass surgery? Can a mortal human being cope daily with the emotional stress and technical demands of this operation without a deep and abiding conviction that this treatment has great value? And would not this enthusiasm be shared by many survivors of this painful medical ordeal? This is the terrible price paid for rushing new treatments into practice without adequate testing. It is not just a theoretical question of weighing the lives lost by a treatment proved ineffective against the lives saved by the quickest possible introduction of one that works. Lost forever is the opportunity for a dispassionate judgment by persons without a professional, financial, or emotional stake in the treatment.

Examined in this light, it was therefore not surprising that the most prominent critics of the Veterans Administration Cooperative Trial were surgeons and cardiologists deeply involved with bypass surgery. And the faults found were not in the surgical procedure itself, but in how the trial was conducted: The results were analyzed too soon. The surgical mortality was too high. The medically managed patients weren't typical, and did unexpectedly well. More bypass grafts should have been used. Not enough of the grafts remained fully open and supplying blood.

Nevertheless, the Veterans Administration trial left one important finding favoring bypass surgery. A subgroup of ninety patients had an unusually severe form of coronary artery disease, an obstruction in the left main coronary artery. The left main, a stubby artery about the diameter of the little finger but an inch or less long, supplies most of the blood for the left ventricle.* And although the numbers of patients were small, and the operative mortality high, the group of patients getting surgery were less likely to die.

However, this severe condition is sufficiently rare that bypass surgery still had no beneficial effect on the life expectancy of seven out of eight patients in the trial.

The Veterans Administration Cooperative Study neither settled the issue nor slowed the growth of bypass surgery. But it greatly magnified both the professional interest and the stakes in a second major randomized clinical trial. This one was sponsored by the National Heart, Lung, and Blood Institute, and was called the Coronary Artery Surgery Study, or CASS. The participating medical schools included some of the most important names in cardiology and heart surgery. So it included Harvard, Yale, Stanford, Duke, the University of Washington (where Cobb did his early experiments on internal mammary ligation), and the University of Alabama at Birmingham, where bypass pioneer John W. Kirklin operated.

---

*The layout of coronary arteries varies somewhat among individuals, and in about 10 percent of the cases the right coronary artery plays a more important role.

There were solid reasons to believe that CASS would succeed where the Veterans study had failed, and demonstrate concrete benefits of bypass surgery beyond relief of angina. The quality of the surgery in the Veterans trial had drawn criticism; the CASS study included some of the nation's biggest names in academic medicine. Moreover, heart surgeons believed that improved methods of protecting the heart during the operation had substantially lowered the risks of the procedure, perhaps by as much as 50 percent. That advance was of great importance, since one key reason for the failure of the Veterans trial was that 5.6 percent of the surgical group had died immediately as a result of the operation, and those early deaths heavily influenced the survival calculations. While the Veterans study had measured only mortality, the CASS experimenters were also including another important potential benefit of bypass surgery—protection against heart attacks that weren't fatal. The more frequent non-fatal heart attacks provided a more sensitive measure of the potential benefits of increasing the blood supply to the heart. Although the study was launched in 1975, before the results of the Veterans study were known, the first CASS results were not published until 1983, and even then would trigger a new controversy. In the meantime bypass surgery continued its rapid growth.

The CASS study squarely hit its first target, demonstrating how safely bypass surgery could now be performed, at least in the hands of some of the best heart surgeons in the country. Among the 357 patients in the bypass surgery group just five died from the operation, a 1.4 percent mortality rate. This was not only a vastly improved safety record, it also meant that the subsequent survival and heart attack calculations would more accurately reflect the benefits of a successful operation, and not be so heavily influenced by the deadly risks of an unsuccessful one. The CASS surgeons also remedied a second technical criticism of the Veterans study—that too many bypass grafts became rapidly blocked, thus nullifying the benefit of the operation. After the operation 97 percent of the surviving CASS patients had at least one graft open, compared to 88 percent in the Veterans study.

None of this helped. The CASS investigators reported that those assigned to the medical treatment group were just as likely to survive for the next five years as those in the surgical group. Nor did bypass surgery demonstrate the slightest ability to prevent heart attacks. At the end of five years 88 percent of those medically treated were free of heart attacks, compared to 86 percent in the surgical group. For a second time an elaborate and expensive clinical trial had failed to demonstrate the benefits of prolonged life that an ever-growing number of cardiologists and heart surgeons were absolutely certain must exist.

Once again, the debate focused mainly on perceived defects in the CASS study, not in the procedure itself. But this time there was no outcry against the surgeons; it was the patients who were to blame. From Houston, surgeon Michael DeBakey charged that the CASS study didn't show any benefits from bypass surgery because the wrong patients were selected. Those with obstructions of the left main coronary artery were omitted, and those were the patients who benefited in the Veterans study. Other severely ill patients were not selected for CASS, but still sent to bypass surgery anyway. And almost a third of the patients initially assigned to the medically managed group later changed their minds and asked for surgery. Even though they got the operation, they were counted in the medically managed group.* Unquestionably, the surgeons had a point: the CASS study participants had less severe disease than, for example, the patients in the Veterans study. But the strength of the CASS study was its low surgical mortality, achieved in part because the operation was performed on healthier patients better able to tolerate a drastic surgical procedure. As the surgery focused on patients with more badly damaged hearts would not the mortality rate inevitably climb?

It is plausible to conclude that the CASS study had so many flaws and ambiguities that it should not weigh heavily on either side of the bypass surgery issue. But the many criticisms of CASS didn't restrain the pro-surgery physicians from citing some of the apparent benefits of bypass surgery shown in the study. More than eight out of ten of those who got bypass surgery experienced fewer chest pains; they could tolerate more exercise and reported an improved quality of life.

Bypass surgery, like other operations now long abandoned, effectively relieved angina pains. It still made better physiological sense than the

---

*However, the survival rates of the two groups were so similar that it didn't matter in which group the crossovers were counted.

Beck procedure or the internal mammary implant. But the most important benefits of bypass surgery—preventing heart attacks or prolonging life—had not been demonstrated in broad-scale objective scientific trials. But an ever larger segment of the medical community grew increasingly unwilling to admit it. Instead, they attempted to reinterpret the results of the trials, to revise history.

In terms of underlying logic, a randomized clinical trial greatly resembles a football game. We intuitively understand that a football game represents the interplay between complex opposing forces, and involves thousands of complicated interactions between players. Sheer luck is regularly a factor in the outcome of a football game. Did the quarterback's foot slip on an unimportant play called back for a penalty or just before attempting to hurl the touchdown pass? Nevertheless, we accept the final score as a legitimate measure of the outcome of the contest. The trial is sufficiently long. It is played according to specific rules announced in advance. It allows for chance occurrences and unmeasured interactions that may not be fully observed nor completely understood. But only one outcome has any real importance and that is the final score for the entire game. The same rule applies equally to clinical trials, but it was violated with increasing and alarming frequency.

The first trial to be reinterpreted was the Veterans Administration study. Several years after the fact the investigators proposed this idea: If they could discard the results of three of the ten centers that had participated, the trial would then show that bypass surgery prolonged the life of another large group of patients, those with obstructions in three vessels. Three of the centers had experienced a much higher operative mortality rate than the others, so it was perfectly clear why the investigators wanted to exclude them. But this was just like trying to rescore the results of last Sunday's football game after ignoring the three fumbles. It was an interesting exercise but it didn't prove anything.

Next, investigators wanted to massage the results of a European trial so it would confirm the key Veterans study conclusion that at least those with obstructions in the left main coronary artery benefited from the operation. The condition is sufficiently rare that there were only fifty-nine such cases among the 767 participants in the European Coronary Surgery Study. The laws of statistics say that there would have to be large differences in so few patients to reach any valid conclusion, and differences of that magnitude had not occurred. The equivalent in football is the intuitive understanding that any one three-minute period of the game is probably not a valid indication of the outcome. Nevertheless American experts claimed the European study confirmed the one positive finding of the Veterans study.

In addition to revising history the proponents of bypass surgery also had one bona fide winner. Without any resort to tiny subgroups of patients selected after the fact, the European Coronary Surgery Study reported that overall more members of the surgically treated group were still alive. In showing measurable benefits, however, the trial also demonstrated some of the important limits of the procedure. Measured at one or two years, there was no difference between those managed medically and those getting bypass surgery. No short-term benefits can be found in any of the trials because of the immediate impact of the surgical deaths. But by five years there was a difference: 92 percent of the surgically treated group was alive, compared to 83 percent of those on medicine.

Even this best evidence, however, illustrates why bypass surgery is a disappointment in terms of prolonging life. It took five years to produce a result large enough to measure. And even then the difference between those getting surgery and the control group was small. Another way of illustrating the survival calculations is to say that in this trial the surgery prolonged the life of less than one out of ten patients who got the operation.

The successful European trial illustrates another important limitation of bypass surgery: Over time, even the modest survival benefits disappear. The benefit of bypass surgery began to decline until at twelve years the difference nears the statistical vanishing point. Both the European experimenters and the U.S. analysts believed they knew the reason why the benefit declined over time rather than increased. The bypass grafts are just as likely—if not more so—to become obstructed by the same process that clogged the coronary arteries. In 10 to 15 percent of the patients the grafts become obstructed almost immediately. The others become occluded over time and many patients will require a second bypass operation, at a risk two to four times higher than the first one. At eleven years, the Veterans study demonstrated a similar decline in benefit. Nevertheless, the European study was a clear-cut victory for bypass surgery. The benefits might be modest but they were beyond dispute.

Why did the Europeans succeed where the Veterans and CASS studies mostly failed? First, the improvement achieved at five years, while significant, is small enough that minor differences could easily affect the outcome. Second, the patients were more severely ill than in the CASS study. And finally, the surgical mortality was lower than the Veterans trial. A later report from the CASS researchers also illustrates this critical balance. A group of the most seriously ill patients who got bypass surgery showed improved survival at the seven-year point, although the gain was too small to be significant at five years. These forty-two high-risk patients had experienced a previous heart attack, had three vessels obstructed, and had been operated on at a zero surgical mortality rate.

A more reasonable interpretation of all three trials together is that to obtain an improved life expectancy from the operation is a tricky balancing act infrequently achieved. The more severe the disease the more likely the patient will benefit. But the more advanced the disease the greater the chance the patient will die in surgery. So one major lesson of the clinical trials is that bypass surgery is a demanding game of picking the right patient and finding a good surgeon. And both, it turns out, are more difficult than they look.

While many cardiologists will differ with details of this strict interpretation of the clinical trials, few would disagree that patient selection is an important key to success. To observe how patient selection works in a world where the research has never been adequate or conclusive, examine what happened when a panel of the nation's leading experts undertook exactly that task in a systematic way.

Mark Chassin, a research physician at the Rand Corporation in Santa Monica, California, recruited nine leading authorities for the experiment. Among the participants were John W. Kirklin from Alabama, Mortimer Buckley, the chief heart surgeon at Massachusetts General Hospital in Boston, and J. Ward Kennedy, the director of cardiology at the University of Washington. Each member of the panel reviewed the clinical descriptions of 370 patient categories. It was almost as if the group were presented 370 patients, each one different, to assess for bypass surgery. Fortunate indeed would be the patient who could get his case evaluated by nine physicians of this panel's standing and expertise. For each case the panel members were instructed to mark, on a one-to-nine scale, how appropriate surgery might be.

When he got all the results back, Chassin wanted to know how often the nine panelists agreed that surgery was clearly inappropriate. In how many cases were the balance of risks and benefits uncertain? And how frequently did the nine panelists agree that here, for certain, was a patient who should get surgery? Out of 370 different situations, prominent authorities agreed on only twenty-nine cases.

Next, Chassin invited the panelists to a two-day meeting in Santa Monica to discuss the cases. After some give-and-take, the rate of complete agreement rose substantially—from 7.8 to 22 percent of the cases. With more generous definitions of "agreement" the number of cases on which they agreed rose still further. Still, the level of agreement is not impressive.

Kirklin, in a lecture he later made to the American College of Cardiology, put his finger directly on the problem.

"One plight in which invasive treatment finds itself is that there are no studies in the current era, randomized or non-randomized, that allow comparison of invasive treatment with purely medical or non-invasive treatment."

Although couched in medical jargon, Kirklin's point is plain. The problem here is not the one commonly supposed—that each patient is so unique and his problems so complex that interpretation is difficult. The problem is that even the best experts do not have adequate scientific studies on which to base a sound judgment. If patient selection was one critical term in the bypass equation, the prospects were no more reassuring on the other: keeping surgical mortality low.

The Veterans study offered the first clues about how easy it was to lose lives in bypass surgery. From the moment it was published famous surgeons were claiming that its 5.6 percent mortality rate was unacceptably high. Later the investigators revealed that ten of the medical centers had conducted 87 percent of the operations at a mortality rate of 3.3 percent. But at three Veterans hospitals the combined death rate was 23 percent among forty-five patients. That mortality rate gap changes the question in a striking manner: The life-and-death question here is not patient selection. It is surgeon selection. The surgical results in the CASS study were much improved, but the same truth reared its ugly head again, even among the medical centers expected to be the finest in the world. This is what happened:

J. Ward Kennedy, the University of Washington authority on cardiology, went down to San Francisco one April to talk to a national meeting of heart surgeons. The University of Washington had coordinated the CASS study, and Kennedy had a massive file not just on the 390 patients in the randomized trial, but a much richer trove of detailed data on 6,176 patients operated on at fifteen cooperating centers who had contributed their cases to a central CASS registry. Since it was undoubtedly the richest and most complete library of data on the subject, Kennedy had the surgeons' rapt attention for his analysis of why their patients died on the table in bypass surgery. There was a learned discussion about factors such as the effects of left ventricular wall motion scores and the degree of stenosis, or narrowing, of the left main coronary artery. Then Kennedy showed them the comparisons between hospitals.

These were not ordinary community hospitals doing the best they could with the people and equipment at hand. These were the medical elite from Harvard, Stanford, Duke, from Alabama and Loma Linda, from the Mayo Clinic and Boston University. But the contrasts between hospitals was no less striking. The mortality rate at the medical center with the worst record was twenty-two times higher than the hospital with the best performance.

But what about differences in patients? Maybe one center took unusual numbers of tough cases. That's the exact subject on which Kennedy, a major authority, had the best information in the world. He could perform the most sophisticated adjustments for patients' differences then possible. Furthermore, he had more than 6,000 patients to validate the calculations. So Kennedy made a second comparison after adjusting for patient characteristics. After adjustment, the patient receiving surgery in the weakest hospital was now thirty-two times more likely to die, instead of twenty-two times. Not only was the weakest center losing patients who would have lived at the typical hospital, the best surgeons were saving patients likely to die elsewhere.

Overall, Kennedy's chart showed four centers with death rates under 1 percent, results that would be rated outstanding by almost any measure. Nine more hospitals fell in the middle with 1 to 4 percent death rates. Finally, two centers had mortality rates in excess of 6 percent. Adjusting for differences in patients only affected the ranking of three of fifteen hospitals. But it didn't affect any of the hospitals at the extremes.

After Kennedy's presentation, a Los Angeles heart surgeon, Quentin R. Stiles, told a little story about his own experiences:

"About ten years ago I was asked to chair a committee to report on cardiac surgery in our Los Angeles area, mainly regarding operative mortality. The variations among our institutions was enormous. Los Angeles at that time had thirty-three hospitals doing cardiac surgery, and the mortality figures ranged from five percent in the hospitals doing the highest volume up to forty percent in one and over fifty percent in another hospital, both doing moderate amounts of cardiac surgery.

"What happened since then? The two with flagrant results are still in business and still having their problems. Why do hospitals continue with heart surgery when results are unacceptable? Ego, prestige, and financial rewards are sometimes more important than patient care."

In the end, that left bypass surgery an operation that carried a high probability of one proven benefit: a notable reduction in angina pain. And it offered one possible gain: prolonged life in some patients. Measured against those benefits were risks far more formidable than usually disclosed to the typical heart patient. First, the risk of death in the operation. The most recent and comprehensive figures available, from California, show 5.65 percent of bypass patients died. Next comes the risk of a heart attack caused by the operation. Information is much less complete on this additional risk, but the best estimates suggest another 6 to 12 percent of patients experience a heart attack during or soon after the operation. Anywhere from 5 to 20 percent of the bypass grafts quickly become blocked soon after the operation. Data on rehospitalization within one year are the most elusive of all, but one study suggested 22 percent are hospitalized again within twelve months, another said 25 percent. However, these figures count many patients twice. It is likely, for example, that a patient with no open and functioning grafts, or a heart attack from the operation, might number among rehospitalized. Even these typical risks don't much help the prospective bypass patient, since in individual cases, and for certain surgeons, they can be much higher—or notably lower.

This left the world of medicine with a marvelous operation, a major technical accomplishment beset by two serious problems: selecting the right patients who would benefit, and keeping the death rate low among all the patients. More than twenty years after the operation was first performed a serious dent had not been made in either problem. But physicians had a dramatic, expensive, and widely heralded solution to a problem that for two centuries had brought suffering and frightened patients to their doctors asking for help.

8
NO TRIAL BALLOON

Cardiologist Kenneth M. Kent is about to undertake a major repair of
the human heart. What makes this attempt unlike many other such
procedures is its surprising gentleness. There is not a scalpel in sight
in this cardiac catheterization laboratory at Georgetown University
Hospital in Washington, D.C. The most menacing-looking piece of
equipment on the small rectangular instrument table is a Cook needle,
which looks like a medium-sized hypodermic needle fitted with a white
plastic collar for easy handling. Nevertheless, Kent will attempt a delicate repair with tolerances measured in thousandths of an inch inside
the heart. And he will do this while the heart is still beating. It is 9:33
A.M. one Wednesday morning, and Kent is worried about this one.
Even though he has done this procedure more than two thousand times
he has good reasons for concern.

Lying before him on the cath lab table is a woman I'll call Tavia
Wilson, age sixty-five. The previous night she was sent down from
Baltimore where she had been hospitalized in the coronary care unit
with severe chest pains. This had occurred three times in the past
month. Even mild chest discomfort can signal a heart attack with its
irreversible loss of heart muscle. But in Tavia's case this had not
happened. The pain had signaled that sometimes her heart cannot

obtain an adequate supply of blood, but so far it has caused no permanent harm. The most critical network of arteries supplies the left side of the heart and the main pumping chamber, the left ventricle. In Tavia's case, however, the left coronary arteries proved free of dangerous obstructions. But in the arteries on the right side of the heart she had not been so fortunate. Obstructing the main branch in the network, the right coronary artery, are not one but three significant lesions, and they are located deep in the artery where they are going to be extremely difficult to reach. That is what worries Kent, even though he is one of the nation's leading experts in a procedure called percutaneous transluminal coronary angioplasty. When not trying to sound official, cardiologists usually call it just angioplasty, the medical term that means artery repair.

"This is going to be a difficult, complicated case," said Kent just before he entered the lab. "That's why they sent her to me instead of doing it themselves." Then he ponders the implications of biting the hands that feed him and adds, "I guess if they didn't send me the tough ones, I wouldn't have any cases to do." Actually, he does a lot of cases, about forty a month. If he were in private practice rather than on salary at the Georgetown University medical school, that would work out to an income of $200,000. Each month.

Back in the lab, Tavia Wilson is fully conscious, and will remain so throughout the procedure. She has a sterile cap over her hair, and is draped in blue surgical cloths, except for a small white circle at the top of her thigh. There she will get a mild local anesthetic. Kent is ready to go to work.

He puts one finger on the small white circle trying to find the femoral pulse. When he has found it he takes the Cook needle and plunges it into the femoral artery. It is about as awe-inspiring as observing a flu shot, except that some blood spurts through the open end of the needle until Kent puts his finger over it. But this begins a long and sometimes dangerous journey to the innermost recesses of the human heart.

Assisting Kent today is Richard Cooke, a tall, bespectacled third-year cardiology fellow who is here learning to do this himself. Also present is Karen Manweiller, a technician who circulates, talks to Tavia, runs the stop watch, and provides supplies. Behind a glass window is Vera Caro, who today is monitoring the patient's vital signs, and operating the all-important video equipment.

At first glance the catheterization laboratory at Georgetown resembles a television studio more than a high-tech medical facility. Mounted on a rack over Tavia Wilson's midsection is a bank of four television monitors. Over her chest, heart high, is the top part of the enormous camera apparatus that can rotate to provide a view of the heart from different angles. At the moment, just one of the four monitor screens is working. On two lines it displays the electrical spikes of Tavia Wilson's heartbeat. Below it, rising in gentler waves, is a moving line indicating her arterial blood pressure.

Kent now takes a short length of thin wire, threads it through the needle and into Tavia Wilson's femoral artery. It travels up the femoral artery a short distance until it enters the iliac artery, where he stops it. When blood leaves the heart it enters the aorta, which rises in a graceful curve and then plunges straight down slightly to the left of the centerline of the body until just at or below the navel, where it forks into the two large iliac arteries that supply the legs. For the moment that is where Kent left the safety wire. Now he withdraws the needle entirely, leaving the wire in place. Next he slides over the safety wire a short, thin plastic tube called the introducer sheath. It ends with a square housing and a cap. With the introducer sheath in place, with only the square housing visible on the thigh, Kent has opened the road that leads straight to Tavia Wilson's heart. And that accomplished, he wants an early look at just what is going on up there.

Unlike the surgeons, Kent does not work with scalpels, electric cauterizing knives, and gleaming stainless steel clamps. The tools of his trade are slender, graceful tubes, called catheters. Just now he has one in his right hand. It is about four feet long, thin, and flexible with a hollow center. At the end is a distinctive curve, something like a shepherd's crook. He inserts it into the introducer sheath, and begins to slide it slowly and smoothly upward.

"How are you doing up there?" asks Kent. Tavia says she is doing fine. He says "up there" because he is positioned at her right knee, and between them is the bulky image intensifier for the fluoroscope camera. There is a loud "clunk" as he presses the foot switch to turn on the camera.

One of the monitor screens is illuminated with a dim view that shows the vertebrae of Wilson's lower spine. Then suddenly the distinctive curve of the shepherd's crook springs into view, as the catheter moves slowly upwards towards her heart. It is now firmly inside the aorta, but the blood vessel cannot be seen at all. All that is visible is the incongruous shepherd's crook, its oddly curved head and straight tube seeming totally out of place against the dim outlines of the soft pulsing organs and curved bones. Then, as if suddenly grasped by an invisible hand, the crook turns sharply to the left. It has just hit the unseen arch of the aorta, is beginning to form a U-shaped bend, and plunge downward toward the heart itself.

The entrances to the coronary arteries are tiny orifices located near the heart's aortic valve. At its point of origination the aorta is almost the diameter of the drainpipe for a kitchen sink, and Kent now wants to lodge the tip of the catheter just in the entrance to the right coronary artery, no bigger around than a pencil. To make matters worse, the entrance is not visible, and Kent is locating it by feel, gently rotating the catheter tip into the orifice. Now, at last, he can illuminate the scene and see what he has to deal with.

Through the hollow tube Richard Cooke injects a quantity of contrast medium, a special dye that makes the right coronary artery suddenly leap out in bold relief. Because this is a critical shot three copies of the image are made simultaneously. It is immediately visible on the monitor. A duplicate image goes onto 35mm movie film. And Vera Caro makes a third copy on a special video disk that can freeze, retrieve, and display any single frame. Using controls mounted on the table, Kent pans the camera showing first the entrance to the right coronary artery, where the catheter still rests. The camera sweeps along the path of the artery as it winds across and down the surface of the heart, branching at irregular intervals. It is not a static scene. The heart is pulsing rhythmically, and the right coronary artery moves too, like the branches of a gnarled oak twisting in a heavy wind. Kent wants before-

and-after shots to document his work, and this is the "before" shot. Vera quickly displays the best view as a still picture on a second monitor. It is immediately clear why Tavia Wilson is having prolonged chest pains, and why it is going to be so tricky for Kent to do something about them.

The right coronary artery twists, turns, and branches across the monitor screen, in the enlarged image about as big around as the forefinger. Then suddenly comes a spot where it seems to be pinched almost entirely closed. It is a tiny hourglass of an aperture, so small it seems surprising blood can get through at all. A few inches downstream is another lesion, not quite so nearly closed, but a longer narrow place. Then the artery turns, almost at a right angle, and right around the corner is a third obstruction. Cardiologists prefer to find the obstructions in left coronary arteries, which are larger and easier to work in, and located where they can be readily reached. These lesions are in the smaller and more difficult right coronary artery and will not be easily dealt with.

Karen Manweiller notices that Tavia looks anxious and uncomfortable. Kent orders three milligrams of Valium put into the intravenous line, and shortly asks how she feels.

"I'm euphoric," says Tavia.

Next Kent withdraws the catheter he so carefully inserted, coils it up, and drops it into the trash. Now that he has completed a reconnaissance of the coronary terrain he is ready to begin the hard part. Now is the time when things can go badly wrong quickly, and without warning.

On the small table beside Tavia Wilson, Kent assembles the apparatus he will use to mount an attack on the three obstructions. The outer layer is the guiding catheter. It is similar to the one he used for reconnaissance, with the same distinctive curve so it can lodge in the orifice of the right coronary artery. Snuggling inside is another tube, the dilation catheter. At the end is the working part, the angioplasty balloon. The dilation catheter is very thin, perhaps half the diameter of a piece of spaghetti. At the end is the clear plastic balloon, shaped like a tiny sausage two inches long. Inside the dilation catheter is perhaps the most critical component of all, the guidewire. This is an incredibly thin coated wire, only fourteen one thousandths of an inch thick. To thread its way through the twisting path of the arteries and slip through the irregular lesions, it must be the precisely correct mixture of rigid and flexible. If it is too soft, it will get too easily hung up. If it is too rigid, or just pushed too hard, it will cut into the soft interior surface of the artery, causing serious and sometimes fatal damage. Now Kent is ready to roll.

"We have our plan of action," Kent tells Tavia. "You may get some discomfort. That doesn't mean anything is wrong, but I want you to tell us about it."

Karen, now standing by Tavia's head, is working out a more precise scheme for reporting. "We're going to use a one-to-ten scale with ten being the worst pain you can imagine."

They have a reason for becoming so solicitous about their patient's comfort. In the more dangerous moments that will follow, the sensation of pain is one of three warning signals that something is going wrong. If the team does get into trouble, they do not want to miss a key warning flag.

In goes the guiding catheter, and like the one before, Kent threads it all the way to the aorta and lodges the tip firmly in the entrance to the right coronary artery. On the monitor screen, the tip of the catheter seems to be pointing right at Kent, bobbing up and down as the heart beats.

"It looks like a nice fit," says Kent. Next he threads the dilation catheter and the guidewire, but stops both at the entrance to the coronary artery. Through the hollow core of the dilation catheter Richard Cooke injects some contrast medium, so they can take one last look before invading the tight, constricted quarters of the right coronary artery. Out in the drainpipe-sized aorta Kent has plenty of room for his catheters without interfering with the normal operation of the heart, and the half gallon of blood that is pumped through every minute. But now both Tavia Wilson and Kent need to use the much smaller right coronary artery at the same time. Through that small orifice, under high pressure, will flow nearly half the oxygen and nutrients for the heart muscle. So not only must he maneuver at close quarters in a beating heart, he must let as much blood as possible flow through the artery while he is working. One of the laws of physics works in his favor. It is possible to reduce substantially the diameter of the artery without much reducing the total volume of blood delivered, which passes through under increased pressure.

Ever so slowly and gently Kent threads the tiny guidewire into the artery. On the screen it just looks like a short length of wire dangling from the end of the bigger catheter. The clear outlines of the artery are visible only for a moment or two after injecting the contrast medium. So Kent is going mostly by feel, and by looking at the fixed-image snapshot he took earlier. The tiny guidewire can get easily hung up. The artery branches often. It winds and turns like an aging river. Slowly and carefully the guidewire creeps towards the first obstruction. And as he reaches lesion number one Kent almost gets into serious trouble.

The casual observer might have missed the moment of peril. As he advanced the guidewire deep inside the artery, the slightly curved tip suddenly began to buckle as it encountered the first and most severe lesion, the obstruction that had pinched a segment of the artery into an hourglass. At this instant much can go wrong.

The guidewire, as it hits the lesion, can knock a tiny piece of the fibrous plaque loose. With the torrent of blood flowing through under high pressure that tiny piece of plaque is likely to jam the neck of the hourglass and close off the artery entirely. The abrupt interruption of the blood supply to a major portion of the heart muscle is the clinical definition of a severe heart attack, and at that instant it would become a race with time to prevent the permanent loss of part of the heart tissue. It is conceivable that Kent might be able to dislodge the tiny plaque and restore the flow of blood. But in the finger-sized blood vessel he would have to find a clogged opening only about two one hundredths of an inch in diameter with a floppy piece of wire more than three feet long. Kent could take a shot at this, but the more likely outcome would be to rush the patient down to open heart surgery in mid-heart attack. Then a surgeon would bypass the obstruction entirely with a graft stitched to the far side of the blockage.

Another unwelcome event at this instant would be dissection of the artery. Even if it does not dislodge a fragment of plaque, the guidewire can cut into the soft, slick interior surface of the artery, called the lumen. Under these circumstances the dissected flap of the lumen can close off the artery entirely, with similar consequences. If Kent gets the guidewire past the narrowest place, he has some tools available to reopen an artery that becomes obstructed. But just now he has no such capability.

Gently and slowly Kent rotates the curved tip of the guidewire, probing for the tiny entrance to the rest of the artery. Cooke injects contrast medium to provide a clearer view. Suddenly the tip emerges on the far side of the hourglass and begins to advance more rapidly towards the second obstruction. Kent passes the guidewire through the next two, less severe lesions more quickly. At last the guidewire is in place, threaded deep into the twisting right coronary artery. If something goes wrong, he has a greater chance of dealing with it. Now he is ready to advance the balloon.

"You may experience some discomfort," Kent tells his patient.

The larger guiding catheter forms a route from the groin all the way to the entrance to the right coronary artery. Now the guidewire will lead the smaller, flexible dilation catheter into the coronary artery right up to the first obstruction. Because it is not yet inflated, the balloon can't be seen on the end of the catheter as it advances down Tavia Wilson's right coronary artery. But a black dot marks the exact center of the deflated balloon, and on the TV monitor screen the dot bobs and bounces with each rhythmic contraction of the heart. Soon he has the black dot exactly in the neck of the hourglass, and will find out whether he can help Tavia Wilson or not. The whole team springs into action.

Kent holds the balloon in place and watches the screen. Cooke begins to pump fluid into the balloon slowly and methodically, rotating the black plastic handle on the inflation pump, his eyes glued on the pressure gauge. Karen Manweiller stands by Tavia Wilson's head and presses the stem of the stopwatch she wears on a cord around her neck. In the control booth Vera Caro begins to record the inflation, and monitor Tavia's vital signs with special care. As the balloon inflates it will briefly create the very condition they would like to prevent—a sudden cutoff of blood supply to the heart. Soon Tavia will experience the first symptoms of oxygen starvation.

"How's the pain?" asks Karen.

"It's a three," says Tavia.

On the screen the balloon can now be clearly seen, inflated like a tiny cocktail sausage with a slight indentation in the middle where it is pressing against the lesion.

Exactly fifty-three seconds elapse before Cooke calls out, "Balloon down. Three atmospheres." Karen clicks the stopwatch and everyone relaxes a little because Tavia's heart is once again getting its proper nourishment.

Another squirt of contrast medium reveals the first results of their handiwork. The hourglass has disappeared. It does not always happen so easily. While the largest obstruction, this one turned out to be soft and readily squeezed open with relatively low pressure on the balloon. They move on and repeat the process with the second obstruction, except this one needs two inflations, at greater pressure, and some narrowing remains afterwards. Deep in the coronary artery, around a sharp corner, Kent finds the toughest lesion of all.

This one does not yield to three atmospheres of pressure, four atmospheres or five atmospheres, and its appearance is not much altered after two inflations of increasing length. They will make a third and final attempt at the lesion, and are willing to risk more indications of cardiac distress. Cooke slowly inflates the balloon to seven atmospheres and leaves it that way.

"We're down on AVF," calls out Vera from the control room, and then a moment later, "One PVC." AVF is one of two electrocardiogram leads, and the oxygen starvation of the heart has inhibited the ability of the muscle cells to transmit the electrical instructions to contract. This shows up as a depressed line on the lead closest to the site of the distress. "PVC" means premature ventricular contraction. Lack of oxygen has now created enough electrical instability to interrupt the timing of the heart's normal contractions. Meanwhile, Tavia reports more pain.

"It's a nine," says Tavia, after two minutes and thirty seconds have elapsed.

"Balloon down, nine atmospheres," says Richard Cooke. The lesion can still be observed as a narrowed segment of the artery, but it is less pronounced, smaller. Everyone takes a break, even turning up the room lights, to give Tavia Wilson's heart a chance to recover.

Kent is almost finished, but on his way out, he decides to take a last crack at the first lesion, the one that was so large but most easily dilated. On the monitor, the site looks impressively open, but Kent wants to make certain it doesn't close up again soon after the catheter has been withdrawn. He has dragged the catheter back and forth across it repeated times while attacking the other two lesions, and he might have cracked part of the fibrous cap.

Again he aligns the black dot at the center of the first lesion while Cooke very slowly inflates the balloon to four atmospheres. Kent gently warns Tavia Wilson.

"We found that the longer we inflate the balloon the better it works," says Kent. "We try to beat them into submission."

One minute passes. Moving with the rhythmic beats of the heart, the balloon looks like a wriggling worm with a black dot painted on its middle. After another minute passes signs of distress become apparent.

"One PVC," calls out Vera Caro. On the monitor the regular rhythmic waves of rising and falling blood pressure are briefly disrupted and look chaotic.

"It's a twelve," says Tavia. Kent asks her to hold on for another fifteen seconds. Vera Caro reports that her electrocardiogram is abnormal. While Tavia Wilson has reported pain off the one-to-ten scale, a team that has seen many such patients does not appear alarmed.

"How would you compare it to a toothache?" asks Karen.

"Not as bad as a toothache," says Tavia.

In another few seconds Cooke calls out for the final time, "Balloon down." Soon Kent has withdrawn the catheters and discarded them, and then unwraps still another, again with the distinctive shepherd's crook shape designed to lodge exactly in the opening of the right coronary artery. In less than a minute he has the tip lodged in the entrance. Now he is ready for the last big moment of the procedure: the after-action picture. The "before" shot, showing the artery pinched in three places, is still displayed on the right hand monitor. As Cooke injects contrast medium, Kent pans the camera to achieve the same camera angle for purposes of comparison.

The difference is dramatic. It can be seen plainly on the screen, and immediately sensed in Kent's voice, which sounds relaxed for the first time.

"It looks beautiful!" says Kent.

"Am I cured?" asks Tavia.

"I really hope so, hon. It really looks beautiful."

Now that they are finishing Kent asks Tavia if she knows whether her husband has arrived from Baltimore. He had been expected just before the procedure began, but Kent hadn't yet talked to him.

"If he was supposed to be here at eight o'clock, you can be certain he'll be here at seven thirty," says Tavia. "Harold's old faithful."

Now Tavia, sensing everyone's more relaxed voice and manner, adds: "Did you know it's my forty-fifth wedding anniversary?"

A few moments later Kent is in the room next door, taking off his lead-lined vest, surprised and a little relieved at how well things have gone. He says, "You know, they just don't go any smoother than that."

• • •

F. MASON SONES had stumbled into a way to pinpoint the lesions in the tiny coronary arteries almost by accident. But the first technique for eliminating those blockages came from a systematic program of development. It was executed by one extraordinary man working mostly alone. His name was Andreas Gruentzig. He was born in East Germany, and educated in West Germany and England. In 1977 he performed the first angioplasty in Zurich, Switzerland, and became rich, famous, and much beloved in the United States. The meteoric rise of Gruentzig and his procedure also provide an object lesson in both the vitality and the perils of medical innovation today.

In 1977 practically no one had heard of Andreas Gruentzig. Since finishing his internship in Germany he had hopped from hospital to hospital across Europe in a succession of fellowships, a medical equivalent of the professional student. He studied epidemiology in London, internal medicine in Darmstadt, then in Zurich, radiology and finally cardiology. At the University of Zurich he had just barely climbed onto the bottom rung of the academic ladder. And in Europe the medical hierarchy is even more rigid than the United States. So he was hardly a celebrated figure in European medicine. But he did have an idea.

The basic concept came from Charles F. Dotter in 1964, but for years no one paid much attention. The arteries of the legs are vulnerable to the same process that creates obstructions in the coronary arteries, except the buildups mainly cause pain and muscle weakness. Operating in the more spacious and forgiving femoral arteries, Dotter had demonstrated that obstructions could be eliminated using catheters of increasing size. His discovery, almost ignored in the United States, inspired some interest in Europe, where a key improvement occurred. Instead of the tedious and clumsy insertion of ever larger catheters, why not just blow up a little balloon at the end of it? It worked, but triggered only modest enthusiasm among European specialists in peripheral vascular problems.

Perhaps the long sequence of fellowships gave Gruentzig a broader vision than many of his more narrowly specialized colleagues, because he saw in the balloon catheter a new therapeutic weapon against blockages in blood vessels all over the human body: the legs, the kidneys, even the heart. He was trained in angiography and radiology, so he knew how to identify the obstructions. Now all he needed were balloon catheters that would work in the tiny, constricted coronary arteries. These he would have to make himself by hand, testing potential materials for the balloon on his kitchen table. When he had created a working balloon catheter he tried it on dogs. Finally, in September of 1977, he used the new balloon on a thirty-seven-year-old Swiss insurance salesman with severe angina. It seemed to work. After just three more patients Gruentzig was ready to tell the world.

While Gruentzig had neither reputation nor an influential backer, he was not without assets. Among other things, he was young, charming, uncommonly handsome, with a shock of dark hair and a moustache that put him in a league with Clark Gable. His dashing continental style was something of a contrast with the more tightly controlled American medical manner, but years later former colleagues would describe him as charismatic.

Kenneth Kent remembered attending the medical world's version of the official birth announcement of angioplasty. It was November 1977 in Miami. Gruentzig was presenting the results of his first four patients to an openly skeptical audience of U.S. cardiologists at the annual meeting of the American Heart Association. Yes, he could inflate the balloon and it would appear to reduce the size of the lesion. But what would prevent it from soon springing back into its original shape, or reappearing through the same process that created it? With just four patients and less than three months, Gruentzig couldn't answer that question yet. And it was a problem that would haunt angioplasty for many years to come. Still, it was an exciting idea, removing the obstructions without resorting to the more violent open heart surgery. If anyone was struck by how hard surgery was on the patients, it was likely the cardiologists who saw them soon after the operation. Or who never saw them alive again.

Something else made angioplasty particularly appealing to the cardiologists assembled in Miami. Here was a procedure they could do themselves. They already were trained to use the catheters for diagnostic purposes, to pinpoint the location of the obstructions. Here was a new therapy that was a logical outgrowth of their training. There was another factor, probably not discussed openly or at length. If angioplasty worked, no longer would cardiologists be primarily diagnosticians who sent their most seriously ailing patients to the surgeons. They might be able to solve many more problems themselves. This new piece of medical turf would belong to them. And so vast were the numbers of people suffering from angina that it might also be very lucrative turf.

The next year Kenneth Kent, then at the National Institutes of Health, went to Zurich. NIH takes special pride in being on the cutting edge of change, and already Gruentzig's idea fell in the category of a promising new development worthy of evaluation. When he arrived in Zurich, Kent found Gruentzig installed in a tiny cubbyhole in the basement of University Hospital. Kent observed Gruentzig perform the procedure four times. Even more important, he talked Gruentzig into giving him three balloon catheters and three guiding catheters. Gruentzig had designed the catheters and they were hand made, so anyone who wanted to perform angioplasty also had to talk Gruentzig into providing the necessary hardware. Kent paid cash and took them back in his suitcase. Now he would try it himself.

Kent was not first. He was just early. At least three other American cardiologists had gotten catheters from Gruentzig and had performed procedures. When he got back to Bethesda, Kent immediately began a search for The Perfect Patient, and also the easiest possible case. It would be much too dangerous to go after the lesion that was easiest to reach: a blockage in the short, stubby left main coronary artery through which flows most of the heart's entire blood supply. While it is the largest of the coronary arteries, and leads immediately from the aorta, any accidental damage ran an unacceptably high risk of killing the patient outright. But after an inch or two, the left main divides. One branch circles around to the back side of the heart, and the other is the angioplasters' dream: the left anterior (front) descending artery, or LAD. Some cardiologists call a blockage in that artery the widow maker, because the LAD supplies so much of the blood to the left ventricle. Surprisingly, however, bypassing the LAD with surgery had never produced the expected benefits, either in prolonged life or averted heart attacks. That made an obstruction in the LAD a perfect target for angioplasty.

It took Kent almost three months to find the ideal patient, a West Virginia bricklayer with a history of chest pains that had suddenly become more severe without much observable change in the lesion, located near the entrance to the LAD. He invited two cardiologists who had already done angioplasty to be present for his first attempt, but they couldn't come.

"That didn't work," said Kent, "so I just decided to bite the bullet. I was quite honest with the guy. I told him that I'd never done any, that I'd seen them done, and that we had all the equipment. He was desperate."

Since the cath lab at NIH was equipped with an elaborate audio-visual setup, Kent attracted a large gathering. The surgeons, who until then had a monopoly on such treatments, watched with special interest. Kent was so concerned about what would happen to the patient that he was scarcely aware of the audience. He kept getting the guide-wire hung up in the wrong branch, so it became a lengthy procedure, but a success. It was February 1979.

By June of 1979 it was possible for all the cardiologists who knew how to perform angioplasty to fit in one small room. By then Gruentzig had done forty, Kent just two. Add the procedures done by Simon H. Stertzer in New York, Richard K. Myler in San Francisco, and David Williams in Providence, and the total barely passed 200.

Had this been a drug the next step for the infant procedure would have been Phase I testing, to establish how to perform it safely, and measure accurately the substantial dangers of dissecting, rupturing, or simply blocking the arteries rather than opening them. Another important Phase I safety issue was surgical backup. Does an operating room need to be available within just a few minutes, with a heart surgeon at the ready? Or can the patient wait as long as a half hour without suffering irreparable harm? Can it be safely performed in the hundreds of catheterization labs located in hospitals without open-heart surgery? Then would have come Phase II tests to establish whether it was effective in reducing the obstructions and relieving the angina pains. The key question was how long the arteries remained open, and there were fewer than one hundred patients on which there was even a single year's followup data. Finally, if this were a drug, would come Phase III, the randomized clinical trials—the most severe and revealing of medical scientific experiments. It is from here that would come the vital knowledge of which, among the many kinds of blockages occurring at different stages in the disease process, would be helped by this technique. This is the most important question of all, identifying specifically who it helps and who it harms.

However, angioplasty is not a drug, even though it is manifestly more dangerous than many drugs. It is a quasi-surgical procedure. Consequently, none of these studies were performed before angioplasty blossomed into widespread clinical use. Any cardiologist in any hospital in the country was soon free to decide when he would do angioplasty, and on whom. And it would be hard to find a demanding new therapy that inspired more interest, more enthusiasm, and spread more quickly.

In June of 1979 NIH sponsored a workshop to spread the word about angioplasty. NIH proposed that centers who wanted to experiment with the new procedure contribute their cases to a central registry. Immediately thirty-four major medical centers signed up. And as the months passed, scores of other hospitals got into angioplasty without joining the central registry.

The boom was on. In 1978 the cases could be measured in dozens. In 1979 they numbered in the hundreds. By 1981 the numbers had grown to thousands each year. By 1986 angioplasty passed the 100,000 mark. In 1988 there were an estimated 150,000 procedures each year.

Gruentzig, meanwhile, leaped from the bottom to the top of the pyramid of academic medicine in a single jump. His pioneering work caught the eye of Emory's J. Willis Hurst, best known publicly as Lyndon Johnson's cardiologist, but in medical circles esteemed as the editor of a widely used cardiology text. Hurst lured Gruentzig to Emory University in Atlanta as a full professor of cardiology and radiology and director of a new center for angioplasty.

At Emory both Gruentzig's fame and the scope of his activities expanded. He continued to improve the balloons and catheters. He demonstrated angioplasty to audiences of hundreds of cardiologists, making Emory one of the nation's major centers for the new procedure. He cut a dashing figure on the Atlanta scene. He roared about town, too fast said some, in a Porsche. He flew his own twin-engine plane. He was an expert skier. After a divorce he married a glamorous blonde radiology resident, Mary Ann Thornton, and they were graceful and dazzling together as they circled the dance floor. He was given to the grand, swashbuckling gesture. He believed cardiac catheterization had become safe enough to be performed on an outpatient basis. To prove his point, he jumped up on the catheterization table one evening and asked one of the cardiology fellows in training to catheterize him. Once the procedure was complete he leaped up, drove home to pick up his wife, and proceeded to the Hursts' Christmas party.

Then, one stormy day in October 1985, Gruentzig lost everything. He and Mary Ann had spent the weekend at their pastel yellow vacation home on Sea Island, Georgia It was Sunday night and time to return to Atlanta. Gruentzig was the pilot. As they headed northwest towards Atlanta the weather went from bad to worse. A twin-engine private aircraft is no match for a serious storm. Twice he radioed for help before sending a last message: "It's all out." The plane crashed in Monroe County, Georgia, killing them both. He left behind a widely accepted new procedure, and many questions that should have been answered before angioplasty spread to clinical use.

From the start cardiologists touted angioplasty as a safer alternative to bypass surgery. It seemed intuitively obvious that a tiny balloon that gently and almost painlessly squeezed the lesions would be safer than an open heart operation. But was it? The CASS study demonstrated that in the hands of experts, bypass surgery could be performed on elective patients at less than 2 percent mortality and the best medical centers could do it routinely at less than 1 percent. Furthermore, the cardiologists were poking around in tiny, vital, and easily damaged coronary arteries with various wires and tubes. How much did it take to damage the artery? Just the irritation of the guidewire could trigger irregular contractions of the heart. And even if the artery was not dissected, ruptured, or blocked, there was the ever-present danger the artery would spasm, with the smooth muscle abruptly contracting, squeezing the narrowed places completely closed. Yes, it looked safe but cardiologists were tinkering with one of most important and easily damaged pieces of the human anatomy.

While it did not occur to the early proponents of angioplasty to conduct a Phase I safety trial prior to putting it into clinical use, they did decide to keep score. And one useful and important outcome of the June 1979 NIH workshop on angioplasty was the central registry to which nearly three dozen medical centers contributed cases. It was entirely voluntary. Nothing prevented the omission of embarrassing episodes. It did not include those cardiologists who were not so meticulous and research-oriented. And it was not a complete picture of what was happening in angioplasty. But it was better than nothing. And from that registry comes most of what is known about the safety of angioplasty.

From the narrow perspective of immediately killing the patient, angioplasty emerged with a promising safety record. Of the first 3,079 patients in the registry, just twenty-nine died during their hospital stay for an overall mortality rate of 0.9 percent. But it included tragedies plainly resulting from the procedure itself. A thirty-eight-year-old woman died when either the guidewire or the catheter dissected her left main coronary artery. She did not survive emergency surgery to repair the damage. In a forty-nine-year-old man undergoing angioplasty, the coronary arteries apparently went into spasm and he died on the table in the catheterization lab. One sixty-nine-year-old man looked like the textbook angioplasty case with a lesion in the LAD. The procedure appeared to be successful, but he quickly died of a massive heart attack. Still, measured in sheer operative mortality angioplasty looked good.

The results were much more troubling with a broader definition of adverse outcomes. About one out of five patients suffered a complication from angioplasty, and in half the complications were deemed serious. Major complications of angioplasty are death, a heart attack, or an accident serious enough to require emergency bypass surgery, most often because the artery was dissected or blocked. The most frequent adverse outcome was emergency surgery, occurring in 6.8 percent of the cases. Not only were the deaths more likely to occur in this group but 40 percent experienced irreversible damage to the heart, either from the angioplasty, the surgery, or both.

"It keeps you humble," said Kent. "We had more than two hundred consecutive patients without taking one to surgery. Then within a couple of weeks we had two. Both were young and had an uncomplicated procedure." Among less severe complications the most frequent was a prolonged episode of chest pain—the classic symptoms of a heart attack—but without clinical evidence that heart tissue was in fact destroyed. This was experienced by more than one out of ten angioplasty patients. In all, these were far from trivial risks even in the hands of top cardiologists in leading medical centers with a major scientific interest in the procedure. But risks by themselves mean little until compared with the benefits.

The cardiologists provided themselves with a generous description of success. If the obstructions could be reduced in size by 20 percent, and remained so while the patient was in the cath lab, and without otherwise permanently harming him, this was judged a clinical success.* But this was all quite approximate, and left to the judgment of the angioplaster or an assistant preparing the reports. As one investigator bluntly put it, "No quality control was attempted." Even with such a lenient definition the investigators failed in nearly one out of three cases.

When Gruentzig presented his first four patients skeptics immedi-

---

*Later the definition was refined to require also that the dilated lesion obstruct no more than 50 percent of the diameter of the artery.

ately wanted to know why the dilated lesions would not soon recur. The mechanisms by which obstructions form in the coronary arteries remained largely a mystery. Why angioplasty could permanently dilate the lesions—many of which were hard, fibrous structures that had invaded the smooth muscle of the arteries—was just as much an enigma. The evidence mounted that in an alarming number of cases the obstructions indeed recurred within a few months. The medical term was restenosis, and it was to trigger much debate and substantial research. Within six months restenosis had occurred in 30 percent of the patients with successful angioplasty. If one counted only the patients who complained that chest pains had returned, or had positive exercise stress tests, the figure would be only half that size. The mechanisms of pain relief are no better understood in angioplasty than bypass surgery, and so in roughly half the restenosis cases the lesions returned but the symptoms did not. There were two ways to deal with restenosis: another angioplasty or coronary bypass surgery. Thus, any calculation of the advantages of angioplasty had to include the unfortunate fact that it failed in one out of three cases, and that even among its successes nearly one out of three required a second procedure within six months. When all these probabilities were combined angioplasty emerged looking like not a miracle cure but a 50 percent solution. That is, the typical patient had slightly better than a fifty/fifty chance of emerging free of symptoms without dying, experiencing a heart attack, requiring emergency bypass surgery, or an additional procedure. As the years passed more experience and better catheters and guidewires tended to improve the failure rate, at least among the medical centers that had joined the original registry. But the restenosis problem and overall mortality remained largely unchanged.

To ask how angioplasty stacks up against the alternatives, bypass surgery and medical management, is to plunge deep into the void of the unknown. A cardiologist at the Mayo Clinic, Emilio R. Guiliani, put the facts quite simply: "The most fundamental question has not been asked. Does a patient benefit from coronary angioplasty in comparison with current available therapeutic regimens?" Peter C. Block of Harvard University was equally forthright: "I don't think anyone has any data on which they can base a statement that angioplasty prolongs life. I don't know anybody who is a responsible investigator who is doing angioplasty to prolong life." In 1988 the heart institute launched a trial that was expected to provide some limited but objective comparisons between the two procedures by the mid-1990s.

Clear evidence did emerge on one factor that created a measurable difference between success and failure in angioplasty: the experience of the cardiologist. For example, the registry cases showed that cardiologists doing their first fifty procedures failed 45 percent of the time. But after 150 cases the failure rate had dropped to 25 percent. Another analysis placed experience as the second most important factor associated with a failed angioplasty, surpassed only by the presence of hardened calcium deposits in the lesions.

The early pioneers such as Kent had no alternative but to experiment on consenting patients. But as angioplasty spread into broad clinical use the medical world was treated to the spectacle of thousands of cardiologists teaching themselves how to perform angioplasty on the patients at hand. Literally thousands trouped through Emory to watch Gruentzig. Others could pick up the skill from observing or assisting a colleague. Not only were there no formal training programs or standards to insure competence, other critical pieces of machinery were entirely missing. For example, for many years the heart surgeons had established procedures for the systematic review of complications and operative deaths. As later chapters of this book will show, the system frequently looks better on paper than it works in practice. But at least the surgeons had a system. The cardiologists had nothing. After years of delay the American College of Cardiology and the American Heart Association joined to issue an advisory recommendation on training. Before undertaking angioplasty without supervision a cardiologist ought to have performed 125 procedures, including at least seventy-five as the primary operator. In a bow to the practicing cardiologists unlikely to return to school for such extended training, the task force suggested the experienced physician could gain acceptable experience with fifty cases in a "tutorial setting." But the same document conceded such standards were not being widely observed:

"It is recognized that hospitals are under intense pressure to grant privileges to cardiologists who have not had adequate training so as to protect the hospitals' referral base. This practice should not be condoned. . . ."

So thus it happened that angioplasty propelled cardiology into the big leagues with heart surgery, where small mistakes could lead to major complications or death. They had developed a promising new treatment, and were perfecting it with each passing year. What cardiology lacked was the proper testing, structure, safety standards, and quality assurance programs to protect patients from the new dangers to which they were being exposed daily in ever-increasing numbers.

• • •

WHY DID ANGIOPLASTY grow so quickly? One powerful propelling force was a topic most physicians prefer not to discuss in polite society. It was the money. Rarely had a new medical procedure come along that was quite so lucrative while remaining so free of restraints on potential excesses. Consider its impact on the economic status of cardiologists:

Cardiology is part of the formal medical specialty of internal medicine. In the most recent year for which data are available, 1986, average annual income in the specialty was $109,400, trailing well behind surgeons, who earned $162,400. Specific figures are not available, but it is likely that cardiologists who do not perform angioplasty typically earn more than a majority of their colleagues in internal medicine, but less than the typical surgeon. Now enter angioplasty.

A typical fee for angioplasty in 1988 was $5,000. To maintain their skills, the American College of Cardiology recommends that its qualified members perform at least one angioplasty procedure each week. Therefore, a cardiologist who just slightly exceeded the bare minimum, doing two procedures a week, would increase his annual earnings by an additional $520,000. Even allowing for those who charge substantially lower fees, angioplasty offers powerful financial incentives. Such fees are not unprecedented in medicine, and are comparable to heart surgeons and neurosurgeons. But nowhere else in medicine are such powerful financial incentives combined with absence of the checks and balances achieved through the referral system.

It is a standing joke in medicine that surgeons find many more patients who would benefit from surgery than do other physicians. The truth underlying the humor has been demonstrated in numerous studies showing a strong relationship between the number of surgeons who know how to perform a certain operation in a community and the likelihood it will be performed. Income is only one ingredient in the specialists' understandable enthusiasm for the exercise of their skills. But a surgeon must depend on referrals, and a second physician without personal or financial involvement in the treatment must generally agree the patient will benefit. It had been, in fact, the cardiologists who were the gatekeepers for open heart surgery. They identified possible candidates and if the surgery was ineffective, they would be the first to know. Angioplasty changed that relationship.

Into cardiologists' offices across the land came an unending parade of patients with two of the most common serious ailments in medicine: chest pains or a recent heart attack. Robert Reis, a Miami heart surgeon who operated at NIH, describes what happens next: "There is a real problem with the system here. You have the person who is doing the diagnostic studies, recommending and then performing therapy, and then evaluating the results of therapy, and finally tabulating the frequency of complications from the treatment. That's a pretty closed loop."

The primary danger here may not be physicians who knowingly let their pocketbook influence their medical judgment. The most serious problem is unconscious bias of which the most scrupulous physician may be entirely unaware. The legendary demonstration of the phenomenon occurred many years ago in New York City. In 1934, 400 young patients were sent to New York City school physicians, who were asked to select those who needed their tonsils out. They identified 45 percent of the patients. The remaining children who were not recommended for a tonsillectomy were sent to another group of physicians. This time 46 percent were identified as needing their tonsils removed. The process was repeated until only sixty-five children remained who were not recommended for the operation. If the unconscious bias to treat can be demonstrated among physicians with no economic stake in the operation, what are the additional effects of a powerful financial incentive? Kent describes the equivalent in cardiology in modern terms:

"There are procedures going to be done with sort of a Mt. Everest approach. There are going to be lesions that are dilated just because they're there, rather than having any important impact on the health of the patient." Harvard's Block puts it this way:

"What we're seeing in certain parts of the United States is an enormous explosion in use of angioplasty. More than half the patients diagnosed by angiography end up having some kind of therapy that starts with angioplasty. At the same time we're seeing an exploding number of centers that are doing angioplasty, and more and more physicians depend on angioplasty for their livelihood, and I'm troubled by that if the patients are self-referred."

If the Korean war autopsy studies are any indication, it is likely that a majority of the adult population has some lesions in their coronary arteries by mid-life. More than 1.5 million persons a year are admitted to hospitals with symptoms of coronary heart disease. The present annual volume of 150,000 procedures represents a tiny fraction of the millions who may ultimately be exposed to a procedure with substantial risks and inadequately documented benefits.

· · ·

BESIDES ITS SEEMING gentleness, another important difference separates angioplasty from bypass surgery. By the late 1980s bypass surgery was a stable and mature procedure. Significant improvements had occurred in the 1970s, the most notable being better protection for the heart during the operation. But other than more widespread use of the internal mammary arteries, bypass surgery evolved little during the 1980s. In contrast, angioplasty was a bubbling cauldron of innovation, research, and change. There were advanced catheters capable of reaching more deeply into the coronary arteries and new digital video equipment for a sharper view of the arteries themselves. The problem of restenosis was being attacked with approaches that ranged from tiny wire implants in the arteries to dietary supplements of a substance resembling fish oil. In the experimental phase were new devices to assault the toughest and most resistant lesions with laser-heated probes and tiny rotating turbine blades. And some visionaries foresaw the day when clearing the coronary arteries of obstructions would become a routine preventative treatment like having one's teeth cleaned. But whether these potential technological wonders of the future would be introduced in a safer and more rational manner than previous advances remained an important question to which there were no reassuring answers.

9

A MIRROR
FOR MEDICINE

The patient had passed his last medical checkup with flying colors. Since a case of dysentery in the Philippines more than twenty-five years earlier, the most serious threat to his health had been an occasional cold or the flu. Just one week shy of his sixty-fifth birthday he was vigorous enough to play eighteen holes of golf before lunch, and then nine more before dinner. Between rounds at the Cherry Hills Country Club near Denver he had eaten a hamburger with two slices of raw onion. The first sign of trouble came as he played his twenty-sixth hole. He thought it was indigestion. But after dinner at the home of his mother-in-law, Mrs. John F. Doud, the indigestion was worse still. Then at 2:45 A.M. Saturday morning he called out for help, wracked by severe chest pains. He was Dwight D. Eisenhower, the president of the United States. It was September 26, 1955, and he was experiencing a heart attack.

What happened next would make a modern cardiologist cringe, and provoked comment even in 1955. The president's personal physician, Major General Howard Snyder, was summoned. After a brief examination he gave Eisenhower two shots of morphine at half-hour intervals to relieve the stabbing chest pains, and sent him back to bed without further treatment. It was not until 1:00 P.M. the next day that he took an electrocardiogram, the diagnostic test most likely to show whether his patient's heart had suffered damage. Then and only then was Eisenhower helped to a car and driven to Fitzsimmons Army Hospital for treatment. Later the reporters covering the president's six-week Denver vacation would complain they were misled for more than twelve hours into believing the president's condition was nothing more than indigestion. In retrospect it seems likely that the president's physicians did not immediately identify the heart attack with enough confidence to make an announcement. Probably they were only concealing their uncertainty.

The most important citizen of the United States was suffering from a major threat to his life. A famous cardiologist, Paul Dudley White, was rushed from Boston to Denver, the only passenger on a four-engine Air Force plane. He immediately examined the president. He found Eisenhower's temperature slightly elevated, 99°F. His pulse was somewhat rapid, ninety-two beats a minute, compared to a normal seventy-two, and his blood pressure was slightly lower than normal. All this suggested a heart under stress but still performing reliably. Eisenhower's white blood cell count was somewhat elevated, which was also consistent, since white blood cells go to work on any area of dead or damaged tissue, including the heart. The key evidence came from his electrocardiogram, which maps out the pattern of the electrical signals as they are transmitted across the heart muscle, triggering the carefully timed contraction of the heart. On the president's electrocardiogram White found the unmistakable electrical signature of permanent damage to the heart. White believed the evidence was clear. An area of muscle tissue, approximately the size of an olive, in the front wall of his heart, had been killed. A blood clot, or thrombus, had suddenly formed in a tiny coronary artery, depriving that area of tissue of its entire blood supply. In approximately an hour's time the affected cells had died. In White's words, Eisenhower had suffered a heart attack that was "neither mild nor severe." It is a description that seems appropriate today. Heart attacks can be so mild that without the telltale signature on the electrocardiogram there is little other indication that slight damage has occurred. And in severe heart attacks so much tissue dies that the pumping capacity of the heart is compromised. Eisenhower was not out of danger, either. The damaged heart can develop dangerously irregular rhythms or suddenly arrest. His physicians were hopeful, but they were far from relaxed.

The next step was to determine a course of treatment. White consulted with the Army physicians and decided on a therapy. It is a useful marker in the evolution of medicine because it illustrates what the best and the brightest could do to help an important patient upon whom the eyes of the world were now focused.

The president should stay in bed for seven weeks. In 1955 about all physicians could do was cross their fingers and keep their patient in bed while the body removed the dead tissue, and non-functional scar tissue replaced it. For one of the most dangerous of human afflictions there was essentially no useful medical treatment beyond rest.* Nevertheless, Eisenhower recovered fully, served an entire second term, resumed his beloved golf game. Not until eleven years later did he experience another heart attack.

Almost thirty-five years after Eisenhower's first chest pains, the heart attack remains a major health peril. In 1987 a total of 760,000 persons were hospitalized with a heart attack and required more than six million days of hospital care. An additional 1.2 million were hospitalized with chest pains or other symptoms resembling a heart attack, but without evidence of irreversible damage to the heart.

The vast changes in the practice of medicine are reflected in how the heart attack is treated today. A casual look at the figures suggests the chances of surviving a heart attack have improved immensely. In the 1950s more than one third of the hospitalized heart attack patients died. By 1987 the hospital mortality rate had dropped to less than 16 percent, and there are reasons to believe it will decline still further. However, this impressive decline is only partly a result of improved medical intervention. The average hospital stay shrank from the six weeks typical of the Eisenhower era to less than nine days, and some medical centers discharge uncomplicated cases after a few days. But a drastically shorter hospital stay doesn't mean less treatment: The

---

*Eisenhower's bed rest was so severely enforced that he was carried to the toilet by two medical corpsmen. Such lengthy inactivity increased risk of unwanted blood clots forming in the lungs, brain, or legs, and would not be allowed today.

cost and intensity of the medical therapy increased dramatically over the same period, and a $100,000 medical bill for a heart attack of the severity of Eisenhower's is by no means uncommon.

The initial medical challenge posed by the heart attack has not changed since Eisenhower's day: First it must be diagnosed correctly. Dangerous though it may be, a heart attack, or myocardial infarction, is remarkably easy to confuse with much less severe heart problems as well as entirely unrelated ailments. The symptoms vary from sensations resembling mild indigestion to excruciating chest pains. To make matters worse, these pains are easily confused with the equally elusive problem of angina pectoris. A complete obstruction in some locations in coronary arteries will produce clear and unmistakable evidence on the electrocardiogram, but in other instances the evidence will be misleading or ambiguous. A series of blood tests frequently, but not invariably, will reveal changes in certain marker enzymes found in large concentrations in the heart. The death of heart tissue releases those enzymes into the blood stream. Thus diagnosing a myocardial infarction is a complex medical guessing game.

It is not surprising, therefore, that physicians frequently fail to identify both mild and severe heart attacks. Medical researchers who studied the population of Framingham, Massachusetts, for more than three decades discovered that one quarter of the heart attacks were not recognized or treated when they occurred. In half these cases the victim did not seek medical care. Unrecognized heart attacks were relatively mild, but placed the victim at the same future risk of death as those hospitalized for more serious attacks. Another study suggests that the most severe heart attacks of all—those which are fatal—are overlooked with even greater frequency than mild ones. A University of Tennessee internist studied one hundred consecutive deaths in which a heart attack was confirmed at autopsy. He found that only 53 percent had been diagnosed. Physicians missed 15 percent of the cases with classic symptoms and textbook laboratory findings; almost half the cases with typical symptoms and ambiguous laboratory results; and more than two thirds of the difficult or unusual cases. "The failure to diagnose 47 percent of fatal acute myocardial infarctions was appalling," noted Edwin J. Zarling, an author of the study.

It is almost impossible to assess a separate but related problem: how many patients are solemnly informed they've experienced a heart attack but in fact did not. The only hint comes from the record in diagnosing angina, where it turned out one out of four getting treatment did not have significant obstructions of the coronary arteries.

Treating a heart attack victim is a little like performing overdue repairs on the barn well after the horse got out. A heart attack means sudden death of heart tissue, and this loss is not reversible by treatment. A heart surgeon who was arguing for the benefits of bypass surgery put it this way:

"At least now I can do something. Let me tell you what it was like when I was an intern in the 1950s. The therapy for a heart attack patient was to walk through the wards and say, 'How are you today, Mr. Jones?' And then one day you would come by and Mr. Jones would be gone."

But in the late 1950s, cardiologists were discovering that sometimes the reason why so many patients died had little to do with the irreparable loss of heart muscle. The distressed heart muscle, in cardiac arrest, suddenly stopped pumping blood. Autopsy would show that the area of dead tissue was no larger than the olive-size infarction from which Eisenhower recovered fully, or even no dead tissue at all. So what killed them? The most useful clues to the mystery came from surgeons in the operating room.

Cardiac arrest was also a fairly common complication of anesthesia, particularly during operations in the chest cavity. When the heart abruptly stopped pumping blood it usually did not simply lie limp in the chest cavity. It quivered and twitched like a bag of worms. A disruption of the heart's electrical system had occurred. Instead of responding to carefully timed electrical pulses the muscle cells of the pumping chambers were contracting spontaneously and chaotically, a condition called ventricular fibrillation. On an electrocardiogram it appears as a jagged, saw-toothed pattern. When this happened during surgery in the chest cavity the surgeon would grab the heart with his hands and massage it. Frequently this restored the heartbeat.

Numerous cases were on record where an alert physician had witnessed a cardiac arrest outside the operating room, had immediately opened the chest with a scalpel, and massaged the heart back to life with his bare hands. And a handful of these cases proved to be heart attack victims. Back in the late 1950s this crude but sometimes effective maneuver was the public symbol of heroic medicine at its best. But it was a rarity of minimal value to hundreds of thousands of heart attack victims. Then better techniques began to appear.

It started with Cleveland heart surgeon Claude S. Beck, back in 1947. He was operating on a fourteen-year-old boy whose deformed sternum, or chest bone, was blocking full contractions of the heart. The operation had proceeded uneventfully and Beck was closing the chest when the operating room team observed that the patient was, in 1947 terms, dead, having no blood pressure or pulse. Beck immediately reopened the boy's chest and began to massage the heart. A mechanical respirator took over breathing. He was given a dose of a powerful stimulant, the adrenal hormone epinephrine. These steps had no effect. However, the team was not going to give up so easily on this healthy young boy, whose main symptom before the operation had been shortness of breath after exercise. Doctors continued to massage his heart for another thirty-five minutes without getting a heartbeat. What the electrocardiogram showed then was the chaotic, saw-toothed pattern of fibrillation.

Next Beck took two large electrodes, connected to ordinary household current, and touched them to the boy's heart. This too had no effect. A series of several more shocks finally did achieve something: It brought the electrical activity of the heart to a complete standstill. The straight line tracing on the electrocardiogram was similar to the pattern observed if the equipment is disconnected from a patient. Then, almost immediately, the heart began to beat feebly, and as the minutes passed the contractions gained strength. Twenty minutes later Beck had closed the boy's chest once again.

It was no surprise that Beck's first successful electrical defibrillation did not immediately trigger a medical revolution. In his report he conceded that he had tried the technique on five previous occasions, and the patient had died every time. Further, he wasn't sure whether the long cardiac massage or the electrical shock was really responsible for the result.

But ten years later electrical defibrillation had become a recognized operating room procedure. Better yet, a more powerful shock could be applied externally to the chest—not directly to the heart—and still reverse the deadly electrical disturbance of ventricular fibrillation. But the defibrillator was a cumbersome piece of equipment. It was mostly useful in the operating room. If the shock didn't come immediately after the cardiac arrest, it was usually too late to achieve resuscitation. And in addition to the shock it was usually necessary to open the chest and massage the heart.

Then came a major breakthrough. At Johns Hopkins University, a surgeon, a resident, and their assistant learned how to begin to resuscitate cardiac arrest patients without the dangerous and heroic use of a scalpel to open the chest. As they reported in a landmark article in 1960 in the *Journal of the American Medical Association,* "Anyone, anywhere can now initiate cardiac resuscitative procedures. All that is needed are two hands."

The three men had systematically developed what is now called cardiopulmonary resuscitation, or CPR. In a series of experiments with one hundred dogs, they induced ventricular fibrillation, and then measured the effectiveness of various techniques to sustain circulation. Next they restored a normal heart beat with electrical defibrillation. The Johns Hopkins team found a technique that worked. The heel of one hand was placed at the base of the sternum, or chest bone, and the other hand was placed on top. Next, the sternum was pressed vigorously enough to depress the bone more than an inch-and-a-half. The heart, located immediately behind the sternum, is also squeezed and pumps blood. Initially the researchers thought the technique would only work on children, with their smaller and more flexible rib cages. But as they tried the new CPR out on real patients in the hospital they soon discovered they were saving people as old as age eighty. The critical contribution of CPR was to maintain circulation long enough to get a defibrillator, and shock the heart back into a pattern of normal electrical activity. One of the cases in the team's initial report was of special importance:

One Wednesday in January a forty-five-year-old man was brought to the emergency room of Johns Hopkins with the classic symptoms of a heart attack: excruciating chest pains that radiated down both arms. While undressing for an examination he abruptly crumpled to the floor, unconscious and without heartbeat. A resident immediately began the newly developed CPR. It took twenty minutes to get the electrical defibrillator from the operating room, normally long enough to create fatal brain damage. But the CPR prevented this. When the equipment arrived the first shock halted the chaotic rhythm of defibrillation. The second restored a normal heartbeat. The patient had suffered a sudden interruption of the blood supply to the front wall of the heart, and that had triggered the ventricular fibrillation. But because the otherwise-fatal electrical disturbance was halted, the patient survived.

Such a dramatic resurrection of the otherwise dead was not a common event in the year 1960. Word of the wonders of the simple but dramatically effective CPR spread rapidly through the medical world. And the implications of this were not lost on a Kansas City cardiologist named Hughes W. Day. But a cardiac resuscitation program for heart attack patients did not look practical in Bethany Hospital in Kansas City, a typical community hospital that, unlike a big teaching hospital, did not have an eager corps of residents and interns patrolling the wards day and night. Even with these promising new tools nobody was going to save a cardiac arrest victim unless the event was witnessed or someone was on the scene within a very few minutes. Day's solution would ultimately change every hospital in the United States.

Day persuaded the hospital to build a special area for heart attack patients, who could be observed closely by a specially trained nurse. To detect the fatal arrhythmia the patients were hooked up to newly available cardiac monitors equipped with alarms. Day had created the first coronary care unit. In the nature of such ideas whose time has come, similar units were created almost simultaneously in Toronto, Philadelphia, and Sydney, Australia.

These early reports triggered an explosion of interest and emulation. The first reports appeared in 1962. Five years later one quarter of all U.S. hospitals had established coronary care units. The world of heart medicine leaped to adopt this innovation with extraordinary speed and enthusiasm.

As thousands of patients were monitored more closely in coronary care units across the country, physicians began to discover new rhythm irregularities on a vast scale. There were short bursts of rapid heartbeats. Gradual slowdowns occurred. Occasional premature contractions were frequently found. The worst of all rhythm disturbances could be recorded in horrifying and conclusive detail: the complete electrical death of the heart, called asystole, which could almost never be reversed. In all, coronary care unit researchers reported finding rhythm disturbances in 80 to 90 percent of their heart attack patients. Some, like ventricular fibrillation, involved the peril of certain death, while others were viewed as dangerous, or potentially dangerous.

The detection of more rhythm disturbances spawned wide use of the newly developed tools for controlling them. For deadly ventricular fibrillation there was CPR and electrical defibrillation. A drug called lidocaine, used as a local anesthetic in different form, seemed to help other rhythm disturbances, specially rapid heartbeats. And for a slow-down in the heartbeat many centers inserted temporary pacemakers into the hearts of more than a third of their patients.

What were the results of this rapid creation of special intensive care units for heart attack victims? On a per-day basis it was one of the most expensive facilities in a hospital. How many lives did they save? This was one of the questions on the table in June of 1967 when a group of leading cardiologists gathered in Washington, D.C., for a National Conference on Coronary Care Units. If became clear at the meeting how much easier it was to build and staff an expensive new facility than to save lives with it.

For example, one of the early units, set up by Kenneth Brown in Toronto, had twenty-eight cardiac arrest victims, but only two survivors. Thomas Killip recounted how discouraged they were at New York Hospital-Cornell Medical Center after evaluating the first one hundred patients admitted to the new coronary care unit. Heart patients in the special unit were no more likely to survive than those getting ordinary hospital care. Killip, however, believed he had identified what had gone wrong. When the nurse observed a patient going into ventricular fibrillation she would search out a physician to administer the life-saving electrical shock. The rules almost everywhere reserved the act of defibrillation to physicians. Most units required that a physician be either in the unit or somewhere on the same floor at all times. But by the time the physician arrived the patient was already dead. They just couldn't get there quickly enough. Results improved dramatically when they authorized the CCU nurse to administer the shock if a physician had not appeared within sixty seconds. Many years later, Los Angeles

Cardiologist Eliot Corday still remembered the positive influence of the conference. "The secret ingredient came out. Give the nurses the authority to defibrillate." It was an object lesson that rigid organizational attitudes could be just as formidable an obstacle to saving lives as lack of scientific knowledge. And many cardiologists would remember later that the real problem in setting up coronary care units was not getting the money or equipment, but changing attitudes and giving nurses a much larger role in coronary care.

The federal government also entered the picture, sponsoring its own national conference to promote the benefits of coronary care units and develop hospital guidelines. However, some nagging questions remained about the effectiveness of the new CCUs. Hospital after hospital had published reports in their literature showing roughly the same trend: Prior to setting up a CCU the heart attack mortality was 30 to 40 percent. After setting up a coronary care unit the mortality was reduced to about 20 percent.

Despite these enthusiastic reports a few voices were raised in warning. These before-and-after reports were not scientific or accurate because there was no assurance they were treating the same kinds of patients. If having a special facility led to identifying and admitting many more patients with mild heart attacks, but at no special risk, then the mortality rate would go down even if no lives had been saved. But the U.S. Public Health Service official responsible for heart disease programs was not troubled:

"We do not have the proper studies for demonstrating the advantages of a CCU. But now that these opportunities and occasions to prevent heart rhythm disturbances have become a great deal more common, we can be assured that our efforts are worthwhile. . . ." With that assurance the popularity of coronary care units continued its rapid growth.

Many physicians in Britain, meanwhile, had remained skeptical about coronary care units. Their government-run system spends only about half as much per person for health care as the United States. Family practitioners are generally more accessible and as popular as their colleagues in the United States. The economies in British medicine have been largely realized in the medical specialties, including cardiology, and from limiting expensive hospital services such as bypass surgery and kidney transplants. While one leading British journal, *Lancet*, had published the early CCU pioneers, another, the *British Medical Journal*, rejected the first report from Sydney, declaring, "It was irresponsible to suggest that all patients with acute myocardial infarction should be admitted to wards in which they can receive intensive care." Many years later after the coronary care unit had become standard care in the United States but adopted more slowly in England, the British reported a randomized clinical trial that shocked their American colleagues.

Surprisingly, the British experiment was not the overdue assessment of coronary intensive care that had never been performed in the United States. In the trial, a general practitioner named H. G. Mather examined a group of heart attack victims. Then, randomly, he sent some to the hospital. The rest he sent immediately home.

It is easy to see why the trial came as such a surprise to American physicians. They had come to believe the perilous condition of heart attack victims required the epitome of medical technology and intensive care to maximize the chances for survival. Here a British researcher had dared to send the same patients home. The results were also unsettling because survival of the home care group was identical with the survival of the hospital-treated group. And, ominously, the mortality rate for patients under sixty-five looked quite similar to the widely trumpeted achievements of intensive care units.

Mather's 1971 study was greeted by a torrent of technical criticism from the United States: The study was too small to detect the benefits of hospital treatment; he had biased the study by failing to randomize a large group of patients unlikely to do well at home; so few patients had died that, plainly, they had only suffered mild heart attacks, and were thus not comparable to those in American coronary care units.

Mather repeated his study, this time with a much larger group of patients, and achieved similar results. And two years later another British researcher, A. G. Hill, also demonstrated the same outcome in a third clinical trial. Heart attack patients did just as well at home. There were bona fide technical questions and other definitional problems that limited the immediate applicability of the British findings to United States medical practice. But together they represented a body of impressive evidence collected with an experimental rigor that had been notably absent in the United States research on coronary care units.

Nevertheless the declining mortality from heart attacks in the United States can be documented without relying on before-and-after reports from physicians who started coronary care units. For example, a leading U.S. epidemiologist, Thomas Thom, examined the mortality rate for heart attacks in American hospitals and recorded a steady decline over the ten years when coronary care units were established. The British epidemiologist Geoffrey Rose observed a similar trend in Britain during the period when coronary care units were introduced on a more limited scale. But neither Rose nor Thom were willing to attribute the decline to coronary care units.

"The possibility must be considered that it might have resulted from changes in admission criteria and practice. As word gets around of advances in hospital care, it is natural for general practitioners to respond by sending more patients, particularly perhaps the milder cases previously thought not to justify hospitalization," said Rose.

But what about those dangerous rhythm disturbances that researchers found in 80 to 90 percent of the patients, and the most serious one, ventricular fibrillation, which is invariably fatal without immediate medical intervention?

"The serious question must be faced," said Rose, "whether hospital admission causes those very rhythm disturbances which it is now so successful in controlling."

Neither Rose nor Thom precluded the possibility that treatment advances had saved numerous lives in heart attacks. The available evidence, however, was not sufficient to prove this. And as the years passed, the specific therapies used in the coronary care unit were subject to increasing scrutiny which raised new questions about their value.

The widespread use of temporary pacemakers was the first treatment to be abandoned. In the early coronary care units as many as 40 percent of the patients got temporary pacemakers, which were inserted in a large vein in the arm and threaded into the right ventricle. By the 1980s temporary pacemakers were being used only for relatively rare and specialized conditions.

Next to be challenged was the value of lidocaine, and its capacity to prevent milder disturbances of electrical rhythms from lapsing into the deadly ventricular fibrillation. In late 1988 two separate reviews of the clinical evidence on lidocaine in the *Journal of the American Medical Association* concluded that there was little evidence lidocaine prevented the onset of ventricular fibrillation. Either lidocaine did not achieve this effect, or the benefits were too small to be reflected in the results of ten clinical trials, whether examined separately or as a group.

The uncontested benefit of the coronary care unit was the success in halting ventricular fibrillation, which remained readily reversible by prompt electric shock, and invariably deadly without it. Such events, however, are relatively rare. One researcher, Lee Goldman of Harvard University, estimated that by the late 1970s ventricular fibrillation occurred in only about 4.5 percent of the cases. A more recent estimate, based on eight separate studies, suggests it now occurs in less than 3 percent of those with documented heart attacks. However, when the deadly fibrillation did occur, both authors reported that the coronary care units achieved excellent results, resuscitating from 82 to 88 percent.

As national concerns about medical costs grew, the coronary care unit increasingly became a target of critical analysis of its effectiveness, and the medical attitudes that had led to its unquestioning acceptance. Writing in the *Annals of Internal Medicine,* Osler L. Peterson of Harvard noted that Hughes Day's and the other early studies "would not be given passing grades by freshman medical students. . . ." Peterson and Bernard S. Bloom studied thirty-two coronary care units in New England and discovered that only about half the patients getting this expensive intensive care actually had had heart attacks. David M. Siegel of the University of Rochester reviewed the history of the CCU in the journal *Medical Care,* citing it as the perfect example of "the uncritical acceptance of technology in medical services." And despite the growing accumulation of evidence that the coronary care unit's contributions were limited, numerous medical authorities would continue to credit them with reducing heart attack mortality by one third. The illusion had become too deeply embedded in the folk wisdom of medicine to be pried loose with mere evidence. This is not to suggest that coronary care units are worthless. The savings of ventricular fibrillation victims were modest but real. Advanced equipment for monitoring cardiac output helped in the management of patients whose hearts had been severely damaged. They are excellent places to monitor angioplasty patients, who are prone to suffer a heart attack as a result of their treatment. But the contribution of the coronary care unit has never been adequately evaluated and its life-saving capacity has been systematically exaggerated. However, just about the same time that the coronary care unit was taking a beating in the medical community, along came an important development with the potential for helping a majority of heart attack victims.

10
BELATED
REVOLUTION

Scientific research is so commonly portrayed as an endless parade of progress that the many wrong turns are seldom examined. And it happened that one such understandable but unfortunate error had a major impact on the treatment of heart attack patients.

In the year 1972 cardiologists began to reexamine the long-standing conventional wisdom about what occurs in the earliest critical stage of the heart attack. In Eisenhower's day Paul Dudley White had described the President's heart attack as a "coronary thrombosis." As White described it to the press, the problem was a blood clot or thrombus that had suddenly formed in one of the coronary arteries, interrupting the flow of blood to an area of heart tissue. This had been the accepted concept since 1912. However, White was less certain about the role and effect of the lesions that had developed slowly over many years through the underlying process of coronary artery disease. The clots that formed quickly and frequently fatally seemed to be entirely different from the lesions, which were irregular growths of fiber, calcium, and fats, and built up over twenty years or more. As more was learned about the lesions, medical scientists began to question the role of the blood clot.

The reassessment was led by one of the most colorful and important figures in cardiology, William Roberts. He is a renowned coronary pathologist at the National Institutes of Health, and editor of the *American Journal of Cardiology*. While cautious in his public utterances, he is known in the medical community for his pithy, forceful, and candid style, particularly when commenting on the quality of the surgery on the hearts that come to him for autopsy.

Writing in the American Heart Association's flagship medical journal, *Circulation*, Roberts downgraded the role of a clot in a heart attack. In a 1972 study, he found a thrombus, or clot, in only 10 percent of one series of patients who died quickly from severe heart attacks, and in only 50 percent of another group. Thus clots "may be the consequences rather than the cause" of heart attacks, Roberts said. What the victims of fatal heart attacks had in common was numerous lesions in their coronary arteries. And he concluded it was the coronary artery disease, not the clots, that was primarily responsible. Roberts soon was joined by numerous others. For example, a 1980 study in *Circulation* reported that fifty-five of one hundred consecutive heart attack victims had no thrombus, suggesting that a clot had "no primary role" in heart attacks. This left the process by which heart tissue died somewhat mysterious. So what had been a relatively crisp theory of causation now became a fuzzy event resulting from "multiple interactions."

Roberts's revised theory was also politically convenient. It meshed perfectly with the dramatic new therapy of bypass surgery, which routed blood around the obstructions in the arteries that had built up over many years, and did not deal with the sudden blockage of a clot. It was also consistent with the multi-million dollar trials the NIH had just launched to demonstrate how to prevent coronary heart disease. Those trials also focused on the slowly formed lesions.

All this was neat and tidy except that Roberts, who had been right many times, was wrong. As a consequence, little attention was paid to the growing scientific understanding about how blood clots form—and how they can be dissolved or broken down.

One of the wonders of human blood is the ability to effect temporary repair of broken or damaged blood vessels. (The home-plumbing equivalent would be if the water flowing in the pipes had the additional capacity to detect and plug leaks.) Repair capability is essential for the circulatory system which is prone to develop internal leaks. When an injury to a blood vessel occurs platelets gather at the site. Next a blood protein called fibrinogen is activated, and forms a mesh of fibrin threads among the platelets. Soon the threads, platelets, and other proteins bond to plug the leak.

This invaluable mechanism, however, can also produce an astonishing array of unwanted effects that range from the painful to the fatal. In the brain, clots cause strokes; in the lungs they damage sensitive tissues; clots frequently cause pain and weakness in the legs whose blood vessels are specially vulnerable to damage because of frequent movement. For this reason physicians were looking for something to break down unwanted clots.*

As early as 1933 scientists found what they were looking for in one of the most pervasive families of infectious bacteria, the streptococcus. Various strains of streptococcus cause pneumonia, scarlet fever, meningitis, tonsillitis, and strep throat. While the main thrust of interest in streptococcus was the search for more efficient ways to kill it, researchers at Johns Hopkins found a strain that rapidly broke down blood clots. Fifteen years later a team at New York University headed by a physician named Sol Sherry had isolated the enzyme and decided to try it out. In the chest cavity of a young man who had just had a lung removed was a large mass of coagulated blood. It was covering a dangerous infection. An infusion of the new enzyme quickly broke down the clotted mass into a liquid that was readily removed. They called the new drug streptokinase (strepto-KY-nase).

By the early 1970s streptokinase had proven its value in dissolving clots in the lungs and veins of the legs, but attracted little interest from the U.S. cardiology community, which remained convinced that clots were little more than a side effect of heart attacks. It wasn't that no one tried to tell the cardiologists they were wrong.

One dissenter was Sol Sherry himself, who had continued to test anti-clotting drugs at Washington University in St. Louis and then at Temple University in Philadelphia. Sherry and a colleague rounded up more than a dozen pathologists who met behind closed doors at the

---

*The clots can also break loose from the original site and wreak additional damage on the lungs or brain.

National Institutes of Health. They showed slide after slide of heart attack victims with clots right at the site where the tissue had been killed. Pathologist Roberts, however, continued to insist that the suddenly appearing clots had a purely secondary role, and the doctrine in cardiology did not change. And with streptokinase now available in commercial quantities to dissolve clots, this was not exactly an arcane academic dispute. Later the editor of a international medical journal offered Sherry a chance to explain the importance of clots in a special editorial.

"I never wrote the article," Sherry said, "because I could never get beyond the first three words:

"They won't listen."

While Sherry got nowhere in the United States the manufacture of streptokinase was taken up by a German pharmaceutical house, Hoechst-Roussel, which encouraged testing of its drug. Thus trials were launched in Italy, Australia, and Britain to test whether giving streptokinase to heart attack victims would save lives.* By 1976 all three trials had been completed. And all three had failed. The cardiologists who had relegated the formation of a clot or thrombus to a side effect rather than the cause of a heart attack were not surprised.

An important lesson can be learned from the complete failure of three well-designed clinical trials using an approach that was to become a vital new frontier ten years later. When a trial fails it does not mean an entire approach is invalid. It does not even mean that the therapy is ineffective. It is perfectly possible that there were benefits, but the trial was too small to detect them. It is also possible that there were no detectable benefits given the particular way the drug was administered to this particular group of patients. And that was exactly what proved to be the case with streptokinase.

Finally, in 1979 a group of German, Swedish, and British researchers reported the first resounding success. Streptokinase reduced the mortality rate by 50 percent in a group of patients with moderate and severe

---

*A small trial in the United States was launched in 1971, but then quickly halted because of unexpected side effects.

heart attacks. The European trial appeared to succeed where previous efforts failed primarily for two reasons: They selected patients with more severe heart attacks, and followed them for a longer period of time. Otherwise the approach was nearly identical to the previous unsuccessful trials. It was reasonable to suppose that a reduction of the magnitude of 50 percent might not be sustained over a larger group of patients, especially among those with heart attacks that were not so severe. The study, nevertheless, was a landmark for demonstrating that at last medicine might have a new tool to help a group of patients to whom, since before Eisenhower's time, physicians could offer no therapy more useful than bed rest.

Nevertheless, the trial results were greeted by considerable skepticism in the United States, some of it justified. Not only were there the doubts about the role of the clot in heart attacks, but the experimenters themselves were uncertain about what accounted for this remarkable success. "This trial does not explain either the reduction in mortality during the first three weeks or the later reduction, which was more pronounced," they said. Was it a fluke? Where was the evidence that the streptokinase was really breaking down the clots? They had not catheterized the patients, so there were no films demonstrating the presence of the clot before giving the drug, or that it was dissolved later. While the American medical community was willing to embrace some innovations with embarrassingly few questions asked, it could come up with a lengthy list of demands for further evidence when unexpected findings challenged the conventional wisdom of the day.

Then, suddenly, another medical controversy had the side effect of reopening the debate over the role of blood clots in heart attacks. For nearly a decade a group of heart surgeons and cardiologists in Spokane, Washington, had been experimenting with a new use for bypass surgery. They were sending heart attack patients immediately to bypass surgery in an effort to rescue the endangered area of tissue. In the process, however, the Spokane cardiologists had first examined the coronary arteries of an unprecedentedly large number of heart attack victims right at the acute phase of the attack. When observed within four hours of the onset of symptoms they found 87 percent had clots. Also present were the slowly developed lesions that Roberts had found and other research had confirmed. But right there where the artery had already been narrowed were blood clots. A few hours later the clots had sometimes broken down spontaneously. And this may have been one factor that misled Roberts, who examined the hearts at autopsy. Therefore, the senior cardiologist in the Spokane group, Marcus A. DeWood, called for a reevaluation of the role of thrombosis in an evolving heart attack.

No sooner had DeWood demonstrated how frequently clots could be found in heart attack victims than cardiologists on both sides of the Atlantic were dissolving them with streptokinase. At the University of California at Davis, Garrett Lee and Dean T. Mason reported one early experience, following on the heels of K. P. Rentrop in Germany. Three hours after a forty-nine-year-old man had shown up at the university's hospital in Sacramento with severe chest pains he was on the table in the catheterization lab. The monitor showed that his right coronary artery was entirely blocked. First Lee tried to penetrate the blockage with the guidewire of an angioplasty balloon catheter. But the artery was entirely blocked and he failed. But thirty minutes after an intravenous dose of streptokinase had been administered the right coronary artery was open again and supplying blood. A long-term lesion still obstructed 90 percent of the diameter of the artery. But the clot that was blocking it entirely had disappeared. So had the patient's severe chest pains and the irregularities in his heart beat.

Lee and Mason had not, however, prevented irreversible damage to their patient's heart. In three hours' time some of the heart tissue had died. But there was good reason to suppose that they had limited the area of dead tissue. Now there were films demonstrating exactly what had been taking place in the European Trial, the experiment in which even the investigators who conducted it were not certain what explained the excellent results.

Medical progress is not always rapid. Thrombolytic therapy became the hot new treatment fifty years after streptokinase's capability of breaking down clots had first been documented, thirty years after it had successfully broken down clots in the lungs, twenty years after Sherry's first experiments on heart attack victims, and more than a decade after the Europeans began to document its benefits in trials. And what really made thrombolytic therapy take off was not the familiar old friend, streptokinase, but a new product from a hot California biotechnology company called Genentech.

•••

AT FIRST GLANCE it was not a discovery likely to shake the world. From eleven pounds of human uterus tissue, four Dutch researchers had purified four one hundred thousandths of an ounce of a substance called tissue plasminogen activator, or TPA. The substance had been isolated before, but in experimental terms this was an unprecedentedly large amount. The year was 1979. Almost every blood clot included a substance called plasminogen. When activated, the enzyme rapidly dissolved the fibrin threads that hold together blood clots. Streptokinase, later research had shown, was itself a plasminogen activator. But there were good reasons to believe that an activator of the human body's own manufacture, natural tissue plasminogen activator, might be more effective. And even with such tiny quantities, the first tests suggested TPA might be the most powerful agent yet in breaking down clots. One year later, a Belgian researcher, Désiré Collen, developed a more viable technique for producing clinically useful quantities of TPA, which he obtained from a special strain of human skin cancer cells, which grew rapidly in a laboratory culture. But the quantities were still measured in thousandths of an ounce. This was also when biochemists in the infant gene-splicing industry were searching for valuable substances on which to try their new technology. If they could clone TPA, they could manufacture it by the gallon.

For many decades, anonymous biochemists had labored in the laboratories of places like Harvard and the University of California at San Francisco, slowly and methodically piecing together the puzzle of how cells use DNA and RNA to manufacture particular enzymes and other proteins. Just as the knowledge, nurtured for so many years on lean academic salaries and government grants, reached critical mass, some leading lights in the field realized it could also make them fabulously rich. So Harvard's top biochemist, Wally Gilbert, founded Biogen, and the UCSF's Herb Boyer became a founder of San Francisco's Genentech.

• • •

In the vivid book, *Invisible Frontiers*, author Stephen S. Hall chronicled the race to create the first viable product from genetic engineering: human insulin. It was a race that Genentech had won, making it a darling of Wall Street, and the symbol of the promise of the biotechnology revolution. Investors bet hundreds of millions of dollars that genetic engineering would spawn as many fortunes as the silicon chip. Wall Street had invested so heavily that many founders of Genentech were wealthy men before the firm had turned even a modest profit. At one point, for example, its stock sold for 360 times earnings, compared to a normal ratio of ten to twenty.

In the otherwise scarce TPA, Genentech's gene splicers believed they might have a billion-dollar-a-year product. Just two years after researcher Collen was extracting plasminogen activator from cancer cells, Genentech had cloned it and was growing it in laboratory cultures of ovarian cells from Chinese hamsters.

Genentech's TPA came along just as the NIH's heart institute was taking a belated interest in thrombolytic therapy for heart attacks. In 1981 a group of cardiologists at an NIH workshop had urged the heart institute to sponsor trials on thrombolytic therapy, which had already been the subject of more than a dozen clinical trials in Europe and Australia. After two more years of deliberation, the heart institute began to formulate a plan of clinical trials. What better way to regain a position on the cutting edge of change than to test the first genetically engineered drug for the human heart? And what a boost for Genentech to have the United States government paying for trials of its product in the research establishments of some of the most famous names in cardiology.

If Genentech had any one individual to thank for this enormous blessing, it was Eugene Braunwald, one of the biggest names in cardiology. His name was virtually a synonym for power in the nation's medical elite. Braunwald had headed cardiology at the National Institutes of Health. He was chairman of the Department of Medicine at Harvard. He was editor-in-chief of a major textbook. He was physician-in-chief of a famous Harvard-affiliated hospital, Brigham and Women's.

In the early 1980s, however, Braunwald's name had also become closely associated with what could go wrong in high-powered academic medicine. One day workers in one of Braunwald's labs confided that they suspected a heart researcher named John Roland Darsee was fabricating the data for scientific experiments. Initially, Braunwald decided to treat it as an isolated mistake by a brilliant young research physician and tried to keep the misdeed secret. But Braunwald was later deeply embarrassed when it turned out Darsee had fabricated his research on a vast scale. He was even more stung when outside researchers criticized Darsee's forty-seven coauthors—including Braunwald—for sharing in the credit for numerous other Darsee studies that had obvious discrepancies, omissions, or procedural shortcomings. Braunwald, however, survived the scandal. Not only did Braunwald have a prestige chair in one of the nation's leading medical schools, he also sat on the editorial board of the influential *New England Journal of Medicine.*

It was thus in the *New England Journal of Medicine* in 1984 that Braunwald proclaimed thrombolytic therapy the new frontier in the treatment of heart attacks. At the time TPA was then so new and scarce that there were published reports of it being tried on only a handful of patients. Nevertheless, Braunwald endorsed it enthusiastically. "Tissue-type plasminogen activator has the potential for use as an inexpensive, easily administered, rapidly effective, and highly specific thrombolytic agent," Braunwald wrote. "Clinical trials have recently been started to determine whether this potential will be realized." And it was not by chance that Braunwald referred to the clinical trials since he was heading the National Institutes of Health thrombolytic trials program.

Men like Sol Sherry, who had experimented with breaking down clots in heart attack victims as early as 1958, were astonished to see thrombolysis being portrayed as some kind of revolutionary breakthrough. But at least the cardiology community was finally on the right track.

Just six months after Braunwald declared thrombolytic therapy the new frontier, the National Institutes of Health's announced breakthrough trumpeted on the front pages of newspapers from coast to coast. The NIH concluded Genentech's TPA was twice as effective as streptokinase in dissolving blood clots during heart attacks. Although streptokinase had been tested on thousands of heart attack victims who were followed for months, the NIH pronounced TPA superior on the basis of 143 patients receiving the drug within six hours of a heart attack. In this particular group of patients TPA appeared to be twice as likely to dissolve the blood clots. Braunwald and the NIH were so convinced of TPA's advantages that they canceled the trial; all further experiments would concern other questions involving how and when to give TPA. Thereafter Genentech would have powerful advocates arrayed among the most influential forces in medicine.

Thus it was no surprise that many observers believed it was a foregone conclusion that the Food and Drug Administration's advisory committee was going to approve TPA forthwith. Editorialists for the *Wall Street Journal* had worked themselves into a frenzy of dismay that the FDA had not immediately approved the new drug:

"We call TPA the most noteworthy unavailable drug today. The FDA may believe it is already moving faster than usual with managing the new drug's New Drug Application. Nonetheless, the bureaucratic progress must be measured against the real world costs of keeping the drug out of emergency rooms. It is hard to see what additional data can justify the government's further delay in making a decision on the drug."

Thus Elliot B. Grossbard, Genentech's director of clinical research, had good reasons to be confident one afternoon in May 1987 when he presented the research on TPA to the FDA's Advisory Committee on Cardiovascular and Renal Drugs. He had an already famous new drug that seemed to provide the first serious fulfillment of the promise of genetic engineering. He had with him Eugene Braunwald, who in addition to the luster of his reputation and experience with the TPA, was going to speak for the National Institutes of Health and endorse immediate approval of TPA.

However, the first presentation to the advisory committee was for the familiar old friend, streptokinase. It had been approved for some purposes since 1978, but now the German manufacturer wanted specific additional approval for intravenous injection during a heart attack. So the committee got the long and full history of streptokinase. They had heard about clinical trials with thousands of participants demonstrating a reduction in heart attack deaths of 20 percent. They heard about dozens of studies showing improved heart functions after the clots had been dissolved with streptokinase, although some studies showed no measurable benefits. But streptokinase had been around so long and tested so thoroughly that even if one doubted the importance of clot breakdown, the hard evidence of lives saved still remained. Therefore there was little committee discussion and no dissent in approving an additional use for streptokinase.

But things didn't go so smoothly when Genentech's turn came that afternoon. Grossbard had not gotten far into his presentation when he encountered a barrage of critical questions from the advisory committee members, a group of experts from the medical schools. One fundamental issue in approving any new drug is whether the manufacturer has performed enough clinical testing to establish what is a safe dose. Under questioning it emerged that in the widely touted trials in which TPA had proved so effective in dissolving clots, the experimenters had encountered an unacceptably high frequency of internal bleeding, including in the brain, where cerebral hemorrhages were observed. So it was necessary to reduce the dose in mid-trial, and no one could immediately say how many participants got the lower dose. Did the success of TPA depend on dosages that were dangerously high? One key purpose of testing is to establish the precise level at which the advantages of the drug most outweigh its inevitable risks. Second, quite deep into the testing regime, Genentech had switched to a new variant of TPA with a different molecular structure and a higher recommended dose. Grossbard told the committee that the two variants were so similar that results of tests on the earlier type were valid. Some committee members were not so sure, pointing out that they were being asked to approve a drug that in its recommended dose and current molecular structure had been tested on only 300 people.

Finally, Grossbard could not answer a series of questions about TPA's effectiveness. The committee members said they were fully convinced that TPA could dissolve clots. But did Genentech have evidence that simply dissolving clots with TPA was going to benefit heart attack victims? Genentech had no completed studies suggesting that patients given TPA were less likely to die, or that their hearts suffered less damage. Later, Genentech would cry "foul" over this line of questioning. Years of tests on streptokinase and other clot-dissolving agents had demonstrated the benefit of this property. All Genentech should have to prove was that TPA could dissolve clots, Grossbard argued.

But the committee members were not so convinced. When the session was over, Genentech had persuaded only one member of the advisory committee. Eight committee members voted against recommending approval, and two abstained. In a last-minute appeal, an undaunted Braunwald told the committee, "I think you have to be very careful you are not rejecting a drug that is twice as effective as the one you approved two hours ago."

The advisory committee's action came as a major shock to Genentech and its ever-growing band of allies, proponents, and investors. The *Wall Street Journal* attacked the committee's temerity for insisting on more complete evidence of TPA's benefits, in an editorial titled "The Flat Earth Committee."

"[The advisory committee's] mindset is not limited to the injunction 'do no harm.' It insists that clinical physicians and the peer review journals cannot be trusted to reach judgments of what works; that the efficacy can only be demonstrated in elaborate and costly statistical studies." The *Journal*'s editorial stands as an excellent example of the ritual faith in medical authority, and the uncritical belief in the value of medical innovation. When the "medical breakthrough" story became wedded to the "technological revolution" story this fusion of two of the most powerful pieces of American folk wisdom created an image so irresistible that scientific evidence became unnecessary.

However, Genentech had to wait only seven months for final approval from the FDA, and so important was the decision that Genentech literally lit the sky over San Francisco Bay with a massive display of fireworks. Two days later Genentech sales representatives were handing out information to the American Heart Association meeting at Disneyland. Seventy-five new salesmen, secretly trained in advance on their vacation time, were immediately hired away from other companies and sent to sell the drug Genentech hoped would become a billion-dollar bonanza.

The FDA had not simply caved in. In the intervening six months Genentech had produced evidence on two critical issues. First, a Johns Hopkins study, not complete when the advisory committee met, seemed to demonstrate that breaking down the clots did indeed improve heart function. Next, Braunwald helped arrange an advance release of safety data from an ongoing NIH clinical trial, breaking the strict secrecy that normally attends such double-blind experiments.

Genentech, however, got another big break from the FDA. Despite a unanimous recommendation from the advisory committee, streptokinase was not immediately approved, and did not get a seven-month head start on the lucrative new market. The FDA did not approve streptokinase until just days before TPA got the green light. A new treatment for heart attack victims that would be called thrombolytic therapy, meaning breaking down clots, had been fully launched.

Genentech now had an approved drug popularly perceived as twice as effective as any competitor, cloaked in the glamour of genetic engineering, and touted as a "revolutionary" treatment for heart attack victims. Given a new product that might be twice as effective, Genentech decided to sell it for a price that was ten times higher. It would prove to be a critical decision.

The new TPA would sell for $2,200 for two small vials, compared to streptokinase at $200. That made it one of the most expensive drugs in the world offered for routine medical therapy. In the first year alone, some analysts predicted Genentech revenues from the drug would top $400 million. And Genentech sought a permanent lock on TPA with an unusually broad patent. It sought and won exclusive legal rights to produce and sell a protein that occurs naturally in every human being. "The patent covers purified TPA independent of the production process used to manufacture it," claimed Genentech. Thus armed, Genentech immediately sued a British firm which was developing its own method of cloning and producing the human enzyme.

A confident Genentech also approached the federal government seeking a special provision that would have the effect of turning its legal monopoly on TPA into a direct pipeline into the United States Treasury. Under existing rules the hospitals would have had to absorb the extra costs of giving TPA to Medicare patients, at least for the first year.

Genentech wanted the Health Care Financing Administration to reimburse hospitals for the additional cost with a special add-on payment. Since more than half of all the heart attacks are experienced by the Medicare population, this step alone might have brought Genentech hundreds millions of dollars.

It was a landmark decision when the federal government refused. "Health care rationing," cried some hospitals. At first glance it seemed to be the first time that the federal government had declined to fund what was heralded as a major medical advance on grounds of cost alone. But a closer look revealed that the administration had done its homework. It said, "We are concerned that we not create any improper incentives through seeming to favor TPA over other anti-clotting drugs." It further noted that if hospitals found TPA superior, it would automatically be reflected in higher costs and higher payments in future years.

The decision in March of 1988 was the high water mark in the TPA boom. Soon cardiologists, a group not normally sensitive to questions of costs, were asking "Is it worth the price?" And as thrombolytic therapy finally became accepted, more and more physicians began to ask about the data. Do they really show that TPA is twice as effective, as Braunwald had proclaimed so often?

A few months later the NIH published additional results of the trial on which TPA's claim of effectiveness was primarily based, but with the crucial new information about the survival of patients over a full twelve months. Yes, it appeared that TPA was roughly twice as effective as streptokinase in dissolving clots. But did this produce benefits for the patients? There was no such evidence.

Whether measured at three weeks, six months, or twelve months there was no difference in the mortality rate between the two groups, those treated with streptokinase and those getting TPA. It is conceivable that TPA offered benefits that were not apparent because the trial was canceled prematurely by its over-enthusiastic NIH sponsors. But that would remain just speculation. Finally, the trial had one unambiguous result: Patients whose clots were successfully dissolved were significantly less likely to die. But it did not matter which drug they had received.

New and more complete trials began to reveal why TPA's proclaimed superiority didn't appear to affect survival. Streptokinase worked most effectively against clots that had been just formed, and its clot-breaking ability declined somewhat with time. TPA did not appear to suffer a similar decline, at least in the first six hours. However, thrombolytic therapy was most effective within three hours or less of when the symptoms began, and when the clot first formed. Thus when measured during the period when the greatest potential benefits were possible the performance of the two clot-breaking drugs was roughly comparable.* TPA remained a valuable drug among a growing arsenal of substances available or under development. But its high price continued to draw attention.

Seeking to blunt concern over its price Genentech announced in the summer of 1988 it would provide TPA free to low-income patients without medical insurance, and wouldn't charge hospitals for doses that were unintentionally wasted. A few months later it called a temporary halt to production of TPA because it hadn't sold the stocks on hand. Next a British high court rejected Genentech's patent, concluding the patent covering any means of producing or purifying TPA was overly broad. A similar legal contest continued in the United States courts. Most analysts believed TPA had garnered two thirds of the U.S. market, but it was a small fraction of the billion dollar bonanza once so breathlessly forecast.

While Genentech's inflated expectations had lost it a race, heart attack patients could expect genuine and important benefits from the United States medical community's belated but now avid interest in thrombolytic therapy. It ranks as the most important single advance in treating heart attacks with its benefits tested in over thirty randomized clinical trials beginning in 1959. The most systematic evaluation of thrombolytic therapy concluded that it reduced heart attack mortality by 15 to 20 percent. While bypass surgery and angioplasty stand as vastly more impressive technical feats, neither treatment could boast such impressive scientific evidence of lives saved. The main drawback to thrombolytic therapy was that the drugs attacked all the clots in the

---

*Furthermore, the performance was comparable for three other less widely used and tested clot-breaking drugs, urokinase, acylated plasiminogen-streptokinase activator complex, and a genetically engineered variant of urokinase.

body, not just those obstructing the coronary arteries. It could produce serious bleeding in 3 or 4 percent of patients, and if combined with invasive treatments like angioplasty, in up to 25 percent. Even when measured against these tangible risks, thrombolytic therapy remained a fully documented, repeatedly confirmed, and convincing gain against a principal peril to life.

11

LOSING THE
RACE WITH DEATH

No pulse. No blood pressure. No breathing.

These were the unpromising vital signs of sixty-one-year-old Fred Forbes as he lay on the blacktop driveway in front of his suburban Seattle home. Unless effective measures took place within minutes, the clinical description of Forbes would soon be either dead or vegetable.

It was a clear, cool Saturday morning in March. Minutes earlier Forbes, a retired ground operations manager for an airline, felt short of breath as he dozed, fully dressed, on his bed. He arose and walked outside where he hoped to breathe more easily.

Although the symptoms were familiar, and not especially severe, Forbes was suddenly seized by a pure, powerful idea that seemed to come out of the blue:

"I need help."

At that moment, he was standing beside the open window of his blue Mazda sedan. He reached in and pressed the horn for all he was worth.

He never heard the sound.

Inside, Forbes's wife, Alice, wondered what the racket was all about. She thought, "Oh, lay off the horn. When is it going to stop?" After a moment, she got up anyway. From the window she could see that it was her husband who was honking the horn. Forbes soon slumped to the ground beside the car. His breathing stopped. His heart was not pumping enough to generate a pulse, maintain consciousness, or sustain life.

Alice Forbes called 911 and told the dispatcher she believed that her husband had had an asthma attack. She did not yet know the severity of the crisis. She made the call at 8:51 A.M.

Within a few seconds the medic alarm could be heard by all three full-time firefighters on duty that morning at Station 6 of King County Fire District 39. Local residents call it the Federal Way fire department, for the suburb in which Forbes lives.

Within the minute three men, Cole Kiphart, John Morris, and Jim Wells, were in their white emergency vehicle. The words "AID CAR" were painted on the side in huge red letters. Siren screaming, AID-6 raced toward Forbes's house just over one mile away.

The Aid Car reached the Forbes's house at 8:56 A.M.—just five minutes after the call.

"He's down. Over there. Please hurry," said a neighbor, who pointed toward a crowd of people in the driveway. As Forbes lay unconscious, his son-in-law, Shon Ramey, was trying to perform CPR—cardiopulmonary resuscitation. He compressed Forbes's chest fifteen times, breathed into his mouth twice, and returned to chest compressions. Forbes's daughter, Wendy, was pulling his head back to clear his airway while Alice tried to force open his rigid jaws with her fingers.

As Kiphart took a first look, he concluded that the CPR had probably not been effective because Forbes's airway was not clear.

The three firefighters' medical training had been limited to the fundamentals of emergency medicine—typically about a three-week course. They could perform CPR. They could give oxygen. But their chances of saving someone as critically ill as Forbes were modest without powerful drugs and hazardous medical procedures that require more extensive medical training. Therefore two paramedics of the MEDIC-8 unit, based in a house trailer parked behind Kiphart's fire station, were needed.

As the three firefighters took over CPR, they immediately saw they were in trouble. Forbes was covered with sweat. His face was blue. His abdomen had swelled up. That meant most or all the air being blown into his mouth during CPR went down into his stomach instead of the lungs. Forbes needed help fast.

Things happened all at once. The firefighters dragged him from beside the car to the end of the driveway to get working space. With long-bladed scissors, they quickly stripped off Forbes's clothes. Kiphart affixed two circular white adhesive patches to Forbes's bare chest and attached red and green wires to snap fittings on the patches. The other ends led to an electronic device the size of a large tool box. It was an automatic electronic defibrillator.

This model could analyze the electrical signals from the heart, and decide whether a shock would help. If the heart has stopped pumping blood for some other reason than the chaotic pattern of defibrillation, then a shock would be dangerous and ineffective. Since a machine could make a medical decision that once required a physician, it also meant the defibrillator could be used safely with only a few minutes' training.

While Kiphart hooked up the defibrillator, his two partners were equally busy. Morris got the plastic airway between Forbes's clenched jaws and attached a bag mask. By squeezing the bag, oxygen was forced down the throat, a process they called "bagging the patient." Wells was doing chest compressions. These actions took less than thirty seconds.

Now Kiphart plugged in the defibrillator leads, and they all stood back because of the expected shock. It is at this exact moment that most people like Forbes are resurrected from the world of the otherwise dead.

No shock occurred.

On a tiny monitor screen the defibrillator was now displaying Forbes's heart rhythm, and it was not the jagged-tooth pattern of fibrillation. Instead it showed a slow, faint heartbeat, not even enough to generate a pulse. But it was a normal rhythm. A shock would do harm, not good.

"It is very hard bagging," said Wells, who was squeezing the bag mask. He couldn't get much air into Forbes.

Forbes's life was slipping away. Defibrillation could not solve the problem. He was not getting much air. Deadly poisons were building up in his body and irreversible brain damage would soon occur.

Siren screaming, the MEDIC-8 rig roared down 191st Street. Two paramedics, Mel McClure and Don Flascher, had a tough problem, and they were moving fast.

McClure and Flascher were seasoned medical veterans. McClure had received a full year of intensive medical training. He could deliver babies, administer extremely dangerous drugs, and perform surgical procedures normally undertaken only by physicians. Flascher, a former Army nurse, was similarly trained, and the two had worked together for nine years. In few cities do the paramedics have the training and the authority to perform so many high-risk medical procedures.

They pulled up behind AID-6 at the Forbes's home and flew into action with hardly a word of discussion. A firefighter continued chest compressions. McClure jabbed an IV line into a large chest vein near Forbes's heart. Flascher began a dangerous and essential procedure called intubation.

With a special metal instrument a clear plastic tube is inserted down the throat, past the vocal cords and into the trachea, the airway leading directly to the lungs. Once in place, a donut-shaped balloon is inflated at the end, holding the tube tightly in place and forming an airtight seal. Intubation has two instantly beneficial effects. It guarantees a direct, clear path to get pure oxygen into the lungs. Without the tube sealing the trachea, unconscious patients are also at great risk of drowning in their own vomit, a reaction triggered because some of the air intended for the lungs gets into the stomach.

But Forbes's upper throat was so constricted, so nearly closed by a spasm, that Flascher couldn't get him intubated. So McClure decided to give him a deadly drug that in many jurisdictions can only be administered by an anesthesiologist. McClure gave Forbes a dose of Anectine, which almost instantly paralyzed every skeletal muscle in his body. As the throat muscles relaxed, Flascher got the tube in, and soon Forbes's lungs were being flooded with pure oxygen.

Next McClure was going to stimulate Forbes's one major muscle that remained in operation—his heart. Through the IV line, McClure administered a large dose of the powerful stimulant, epinephrine. It made the heart beat faster. It increased the capacity of the heart muscle to contract, so each squeeze pumped a greater volume of blood. It also dilated the tissue in Forbes's lungs, increasing his intake of oxygen.

At that point McClure and Flascher had taken their best shot. The first frenzy of activity was over, and they waited to see whether Forbes was going to make it.

It was the critical moment, but Alice Forbes did not see it. She felt faint and thought, "All they need is some dumb broad fainting on the driveway." She moved away from her husband, and got into the front seat of the car.

While they waited for something to happen, McClure learned from the family about Forbes's history of asthma. Next he wanted to administer a drug that would further ease Forbes's breathing. But for this he needed a physician's approval. His standing orders gave him the authority to take rapid action in precisely defined emergencies. If he wanted to act further, he needed to talk to a physician. Over the radio, he reported the situation to the emergency room at Auburn General Hospital.

"The doc said it sounded like a good idea. Go with it." said McClure. Flascher briefly removed the bag from the tube leading to the oxygen mask, and McClure administered the drug.

Suddenly the best of all possible news appeared on the tiny monitor screen of the defibrillator. The slow march of spikes across the screen— showing Forbes's grossly inadequate heartbeat—speeded up. It was like watching a slow-motion film abruptly return to normal speed. Under the stimulus of the drug, and with oxygen flooding into his system, his heartbeat more than doubled to one hundred beats per minute.

One of the firefighters felt the carotid artery in Forbes's neck, and exclaimed loudly enough that Alice Forbes heard it in the front seat of the car, "I've got a pulse! I've got a pulse!"

It was 9:04 A.M. Twelve minutes had elapsed since Forbes's collapse. He now had a viable heartbeat, adequate blood pressure, and a detectable pulse. But his respiration was still zero. That was because his diaphragm was still paralyzed by the drug McClure had administered. But Forbes was getting plenty of oxygen through the bag mask, which Flascher still rhythmically squeezed.

Next came the most terrible waiting game of all. Through either defibrillation or drugs, it is possible to spur a failed heart back into operation. But if they had not been quick enough, Forbes would have suffered brain damage and would not regain consciousness, or his mind would be seriously impaired.

As they all kept watch, Forbes's heart began to race dangerously fast under the stimulus of the drugs. From a low of forty beats per minute it soared to 180. His blood pressure also rose far above normal, and then began to level off. By 9:20 A.M., Forbes looked stable enough to transport.

Forbes did not get a stretcher. Instead they strapped him to a six-foot wood backboard. If his heart failed again on the way to the hospital, they would need a firm surface for chest compressions. He was loaded into the MEDIC-8 rig. Flascher drove and McClure was in the back with the still unconscious Forbes.

They hadn't been on the road two minutes when McClure, who was talking to Forbes, thought he detected a response. Forbes's eyes were open, and as McClure talked to him, explaining what had happened, he saw Forbes seem to nod in understanding. Every minute that passed, Forbes was more responsive. The Anectine had now worn off, and Forbes could begin to do his own breathing. Then he came back so quickly that, stimulated by adrenalin and pure oxygen, he began to struggle with the uncomfortable plastic tube in his throat. Forbes was coming back too fast, and McClure radioed for permission to give him Valium to counteract all the stimulants.

By the time the ambulance reached Auburn General, McClure was unmistakably getting rational responses from Forbes.

"It made a really good experience out of it," said McClure. "I'm thinking we have got a good save. The fight is over and it's won this time."

At Station 6 in Federal Way, Cole Kiphart drew a thumbs-up symbol in the logbook opposite the entry for the Forbes aid call. It was the macho firefighters' version of a happyface, and it meant a life saved.

Three months later, Forbes was in his living room recounting everything that happened to him that fateful morning. In the middle of the story Forbes jumped up and left the room. He returned with a plastic garbage bag and emptied out its contents on the beige carpet.

Out came a pair of tan corduroy pants, cut to ribbons when the aid team stripped off his clothes. Next a torn blue check shirt with blood stains, probably from the IV line. A white sweater sliced to shreds. Forbes began to explain.

"My best sweater," he said and stopped. He stared at this heap of tattered clothing lying lifeless on the living room floor. He started to speak again, but he could not. No words were quite adequate to describe coming so close to death, and then being brought back to life again.

•••

IT HAPPENS EVERYWHERE, every day, every hour. Sudden cardiac death (or cardiac arrest) is by itself one of the nation's major causes of death, accounting for about one of seven fatalities every year. Unlike Fred Forbes's case, most cardiac arrests are a result of a sudden disruption of the heart's electrical system, which creates the deadly but reversible condition called ventricular fibrillation. In the late 1980s every hospital had the training and equipment to cope with this frequently fatal malfunction of the heart. But most such events occur outside the hospital.

Much of what we know about sudden cardiac death comes from the living laboratory of Seattle, where a group of researchers at the University of Washington medical school have systematically studied their community for more than a decade. This is what they have learned:

The typical victim is sixty-three years old, and two out of three are men. While often still described as "heart attacks," no sudden blockage of the coronary arteries can be found in four out of five cases. Bernard Lown of Harvard's School of Public Health calls it "an electrical accident of the heart." However, more than half the victims have coronary heart disease, either the periodic chest pains of angina or a previous heart attack. But ominously for more than one out of five sudden cardiac death cases, there has not been the slightest previous indication of any kind of heart ailment—not even high blood pressure. Thus for 20 percent of the victims death comes without prior warning symptoms. In most cases—but by no means all—coronary heart disease is believed to be the underlying cause of this deadly electrical instability. But nobody knows exactly why. More than three quarters of the events occur at home, with another 10 percent on the streets or in other public places.

Saving the victim is a race with time. Irreversible damage to the human body occurs so quickly once the heart stops pumping blood that each elapsed minute reduces the chance for a successful resuscitation.

Among those shocked within two minutes of the event, 77 percent survive to hospital discharge. The chances decline steadily until, after twelve minutes, survival is rare. If more than a minute or two elapses, defibrillation must be soon followed by the advanced care that well trained paramedics can provide: intubation and intravenous administration of powerful drugs. CPR can buy a crucial minute or two of life that substantially increases survival chances if, and only if, followed quickly by defibrillation and advanced care. But in communities with well-developed emergency medical systems citizen CPR can double the number of survivors.

So help must be summoned fast. But almost half of U.S. communities don't have a central 911 number. This is not a trivial shortcoming. A study in one California community without 911 showed 24 percent of all emergency callers reached the wrong agency; in one Florida county, 40 percent got the wrong place. Even 911 isn't a panacea if the system is designed wrong, and the call must be transferred several times. With a *good* system, almost one of the six minutes available to save Fred Forbes's life was consumed by Alice Forbes's initial call for help.

Although other systems can work, it makes sense to have the fire department be the "first responders." In most communities they have the personnel who can get there the fastest. If the department is run properly, firefighters are already trained as emergency medical technicians.

Response time is so obviously important that it frequently has become the sole measure of an emergency medical system. To have a reasonable chance of saving a cardiac arrest victim, the first medic needs to reach the patient in four to six minutes. Some communities, such as New York City, forfeit the opportunity to save most cardiac arrest victims because the response time is too long. Add the delay of reaching the hundreds of thousands of New York residents who live above the twelfth floor of a high-rise building, and the chances of surviving cardiac arrest approach zero. However, a fast response time is absolutely no guarantee that a system will save lives. It does give emergency medical workers a fighting chance.

Growing evidence suggests that the elapsed time to defibrillation is the factor that most influences the chances of resuscitating a cardiac arrest victim. The newest automatic models cost $6,200, and can be operated with as little as twenty minutes' training. In Eugene, Oregon, an eighty-year-old man experienced an arrest at the Amtrak station within eyesight of a fireman trained to use it. He was resuscitated so fast, and with so little damage, that he wanted to get back on the train.* But rare is the fire department today that has equipped its engine companies with defibrillators, and trained firemen to use them.

The dispersion of this vital piece of life-saving equipment has become mired in a legal and bureaucratic morass. Out-of-hospital use of medical equipment such as the defibrillator is regulated by state law. In most states that means firefighters can't use them without a special act of the legislature. And getting legal changes in all fifty states has been further complicated because some firefighters' unions have made it a labor/management issue.

Rapid defibrillation must be soon followed by more advanced care. Many but not all U.S. communities have paramedics, who, with the proper equipment, provide Advanced Life Support, or ALS. Some cities—for example, Pittsburgh—have paramedics on board every ambulance, and a few, like Detroit, have only one or two ALS units for the entire city of 1.2 million, which makes the handful of paramedics practically useless. Many communities are also discovering it is much easier to buy equipment and hire people than to save lives.

While St. Louis has a paramedic on board every ambulance, their skills are frequently wasted responding to non-emergency calls.

"We're stuck with a system here where if you call and say you want an ambulance ride, we don't have the protocols to say no," said Christopher Ronnau, medical adviser to the city's EMS system. "We have people who just plain abuse the system. We have drug addicts who claim they have chest pains to get a ride to the hospital. We have people who come by ambulance for a sore throat."

If unnecessary calls are mainly a big-city problem, lack of central coordination is the biggest failure in the suburbs. For example, through private ambulance companies, there are plenty of ALS units in the

---

*In the coronary care unit at George Washington University Medical Center I observed an alert nurse restore the heart beat by instructing the still-conscious patient to cough a couple of times. She had reacted to ventricular fibrillation so quickly that a shock was not needed.

suburbs of Tacoma, Washington. But because of lack of centralized direction there is no way to identify which unit can get there fastest.

The medics on the street need to work closely with physicians. While most physicians get training in how to intubate, the procedure is so dangerous that many hospitals allow only anesthesiologists to do it. Performing these advanced medical procedures in the field requires a close partnership between emergency room physicians and paramedics, careful training and supervision, and mutual rapport. The training for Seattle area medics was so rigorous that Mel McClure thought his U.S. Marine Corps boot camp was easier. But few cities have a full-time medical director or the equivalent, a cadre of physicians willing to devote long extra hours on a regular basis, usually without pay.

However, under the best of EMS systems, only a fraction of the sudden cardiac death victims will ultimately be saved. The essential first pre-condition is a witness to summon help immediately. In the Seattle area's state-of-the-art system 26 percent of the witnessed arrests survived to hospital discharge compared to 5 percent survival from arrests when another person was not present at the instant of collapse. At the current state of EMS technology and organization it is reasonable to hope to save from 15 to 20 percent of the 300,000 annual deaths from out-of-hospital cardiac arrests, according to Paul E. Pepe, president of the National Association of EMS physicians. In gross numbers that would be the rough equivalent of eliminating all deaths from automobile accidents, a savings of 45,000 to 60,000 lives a year. But a weak link anywhere in the complex chain of events that begins with a call for help reduces the chance of saving a victim of cardiac arrest almost to zero. And in most communities today those are the typical victim's chances of surviving one of the biggest but most readily reversible causes of death.

• • •

HOW AND WHY did cardiac arrest become the neglected orphan of medicine and government in a country with a demonstrated public passion about preventable loss of life? Airline safety gets intense government and public scrutiny, with a loss of life of 1,600 persons annually.

The danger of fire is a concern in nearly every community. The annual loss: 5,100 lives. Preventing automobile accident deaths is a responsibility shared by citizen groups, local, state, and federal governments. The annual loss of life: 45,000. But much less attention is paid to sudden cardiac death. The annual loss: 300,000 lives.

EMS was first perceived as a nationwide problem. From the war in Vietnam came the growing realization that an infantryman shot in a remote rice paddy had a better chance of survival (because he got basic medical care fast) than his former high school classmate injured in an expressway smashup a few miles from home. Since the initial medical issue was primarily auto accident trauma—rather than cardiac emergencies—the problem fell under the federal government agency responsible for highway safety, the Department of Transportation.

In the early 1970s era of benevolent big government, and with the prodding of a liberal activist in the Senate, Alan Cranston, a new federal program was launched to do something about it. Given its roots in highway safety, it was not surprising that EMS was launched on the model of a federal highway construction program: The federal government hands out the money and sets standards, and the state and local governments do the work. There was much to be done.

Desperately injured people were being picked up by funeral directors who got additional public relations mileage for their hearses, or crammed into station wagons run by fire departments. Not only were the vehicles unsuitable, the manpower, training, and equipment were also inadequate or absent entirely. The federal program solved some of the problems and foundered on others. It produced a useful emergency vehicle design—the box-shaped ambulance now a familiar sight in every city. The Department of Transportation established the curriculum for educating the basic medical worker, the emergency medical technician, and later the more highly skilled paramedic. Somewhat less productively these standards were often etched into the granite of state law, sharply slowing the process of change.

By the early 1980s progress had been made, but attitudes towards government underwent a major change. The public and government officials at all levels began to ignore systematically all the strengths of a federal effort: The ability to solve problems on a national scale, to set standards, raise consciousness, and provide money. Attention began to focus on what federal programs did poorly—and one weakness was a limited ability to adapt a standardized solution to a complicated local landscape.

Saving lives—whether from cardiac arrest or accident trauma—raised an astounding number of local political problems which Washington-oriented bureaucrats were poorly equipped to handle. For example, many areas of the country had flourishing private ambulance services. Should big government and Washington money put a popular local firm out of business? In some communities the local medical establishment welcomed EMS as a new chance to save lives. But in others it triggered shameful squabbles among hospitals about who would get the emergency patients. One midwestern city manager told me he had been forced to abandon the idea of paramedic service for his community because the two hospitals in town could not agree on a common plan. Finally, street medicine was a foreign concept to this traditional medical establishment. Physicians were trained and organized to treat patients in the orderly and antiseptic confines of coronary care units and doctors' offices, not people who collapsed without warning in a driveway, or fell to the kitchen floor. If there was one major shortcoming in the federal scheme, it was lack of medical involvement. As a result most communities made progress, but got something more accurately described as an expensive medical taxi service than as a powerful new tool to save lives.

Therefore few mourned the passing of the leading federal role in emergency medical services, which disappeared as part of the mass extinction of activist federal programs in the early years of the Reagan administration. By the late 1980s the federal presence in EMS had shrunk to a single full-time employee. The problem was returned to local communities to solve as best they could. They tried an enormously varied number of solutions.

In an era of privatization some communities turned over the problem entirely to private ambulance services. This amounted to little more than benign neglect in some areas. However, other communities, Kansas City for example, offered privately operated ambulance service under tightly managed performance contracts with the city.

EMS also emerged as one of the few new government services that citizens willingly paid for, although once again it was a problem slowly solved. In Seattle it took a new state law and a referendum to approve a special tax levy. Cities like Eugene, Oregon, and Monterey Park, California, sold special EMS "memberships." Some privatization schemes learned how to milk private insurance and Medicare for transportation fees. Most public systems charged patients for the service, although non-payment was rampant in larger cities. But where there was local leadership most communities could find the money.

The single most common solution to how to provide EMS has been to lodge it in what generally proved to be an inhospitable environment: the local fire department. On paper it seemed to be the obvious solution. It was the centralized, quasi-military, twenty-four-hour-a-day service intended to protect lives and property. Engine companies already responded to auto accidents where their equipment was frequently needed to extinguish fires and extricate victims trapped in the wreckage. But from the start there was friction between the firefighters, or what are called the "fire suppression" units, and the new medics.

The lowest-level medic—the EMT—required less training than a line firefighter. In many departments EMTs were also paid less, and frequently they got treated like second-class citizens. In one Ohio city the firefighters painted a yellow line down the center of a fire station and forbade the medics to cross it. In a Washington, D.C., suburb firefighters were assigned to drive the ambulance as punishment. In Detroit the firefighters insisted that if not enough medics are available, an emergency ambulance be withdrawn from service rather than have a firefighter drive it. On top of all this the EMTs had to work harder than the typical firemen. On any given shift they might respond to twice as many calls. In very short order this could add up to low morale, poor performance, rapid turnover, or all three.

Here's how Rodney Dreifuss, the St. Louis EMS director described it:

"You'll find it back east, you'll find it virtually everywhere in the country. The policemen want to catch crooks. The firefighters want to put out fires, and they want to leave the medical work, and touching patients, to the EMS people."

In desperation many cities moved EMS entirely out of the fire department and established it as a separate department. This, for example, is the situation in St. Louis, Washington, D.C., and New

York City. But the price of peace is loss of a reservoir of trained manpower that could be effectively and inexpensively mobilized to help those who need medical help fast.

Forward-thinking fire chiefs saw EMS as a key role for the future, for a long-standing public service that was in growing danger of falling victim to its own success. Decades of successful building code enforcement, and promotion of smoke detectors and sprinkler systems had created a steady decline in the number of fires. Serious fires in structures became so rare in the suburbs that the size and future budgets of fire departments were threatened. In most communities about 70 percent of all emergency calls were for the medics.

As the 1980s rolled to a close, the American public remained astonishingly tolerant—or perhaps unaware—of the nation-wide failings of EMS. Slow response times, shortages of paramedics, and horror stories got major media attention in a few big cities, notably Washington, D.C., New York City, and Detroit. But few realized the chances of surviving cardiac arrest were equally low in hundreds of prosperous suburbs, and perhaps even lower in less populated areas. Every day in communities across the country could be found on the obituary pages a report of someone who had died "of a sudden heart attack." There would be little indication or understanding that the nation's most readily reversible cause of death had claimed another victim.

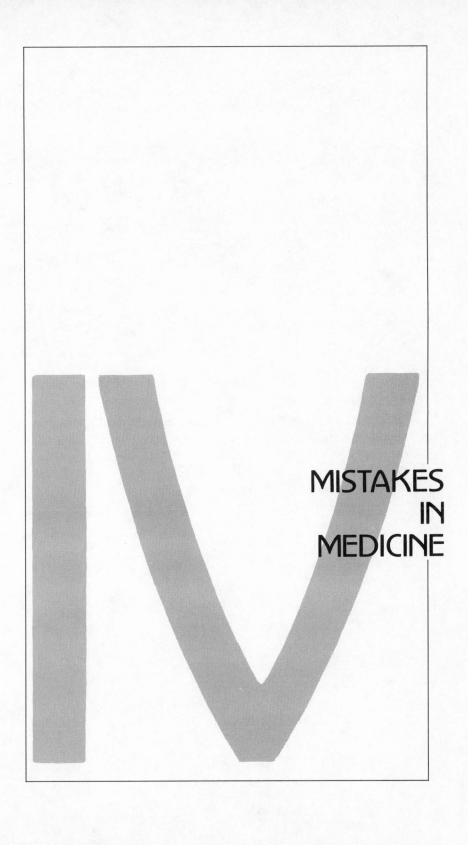

IV

MISTAKES
IN
MEDICINE

12

NO WAY TO
RUN AN AIRLINE

Imagine a country served by hundreds of small airlines, each of which kept its safety record a tightly held secret. Flight safety was under the total control of the pilots of each airline, and their deliberations and actions, if any, were legally secret in many states. The accepted doctrine was that the pilot is the captain of the ship, and ordinarily is the sole judge of what is safe. About the only way to get rid of an unsafe pilot was through a vote of the pilots of that airline. If a crash occurred, a total news blackout was imposed to maintain public confidence. The airlines varied widely in how thoroughly they investigated crashes, if at all, and the secret inquiries were normally headed by the pilot's closest colleagues. Large differences in safety records developed among the many airlines. However, the air traveler rarely got access to such information. Even when accident records were occasionally revealed, industry spokesmen insisted that routes, weather, and aircraft were so different that comparisons were meaningless. Other than paying the airfare of all elderly passengers, the federal government had practically no role in airline safety.

Most of us would consider this a bizarre and homicidal way to run an airline industry. However, it accurately describes the much riskier business of hospital care for heart patients. The many basic similarities between airline transportation and hospital-based medical care make further comparison rich and revealing. Both involve some of the most expensive and complicated technology in routine use. Thousands of lives are at stake on a daily basis in both activities. The two industries require highly trained staff with unusually high levels of alertness, coordination, and teamwork. Both are multi-billion dollar enterprises of worldwide scope. At that point, however, the similarities end and enormous differences begin.

Airline transportation operates under a pervasive blanket of total federal supervision. Every aircraft must have a federal certificate of airworthiness. It cannot even leave a departure gate without permission of a federal traffic controller, and thereafter each new course, altitude change, and other major flying maneuver requires prior government approval. A mechanic cannot so much as tighten a bolt without being federally qualified and he records his maintenance actions on federally approved forms. Every word spoken in the cockpit during flight and key instrument readings are independently monitored and recorded. Many minor and all major accidents are investigated by an independent federal agency, and its proceedings and findings are open to public view. Performance data, ranging from crashes to lost luggage, are routinely published for each airline.

Contrast that system with the equally dangerous and demanding enterprise of open-heart surgery. A hospital can enter the business of heart surgery without federal or state approval, though some states require a local certificate that the service is needed. The equipment, the facilities, operating room, number and kind of personnel are entirely up to each individual hospital, and vary enormously. Each hospital decides independently what qualifications and experience are necessary for a principal heart surgeon, and also determines whether a particular physician meets them. Legally, any licensed physician can direct heart surgery, and other members of the team might come from a wide variety of backgrounds. Also performing the surgical work might be another heart surgeon, a vascular surgeon, a general surgeon, a general practitioner, or an assistant without either a physician's or nurse's formal education and license. If an unusual number of deaths occur, each individual hospital may determine what inquiry, if any, should be made. The principal official record of events during surgery, including errors that killed the patient, is written and retained by the surgeon himself. If the hospital concludes a death occurred because of negligence, avoidable error, defective equipment, or lack of training, it has no legal duty to notify anyone. In many states the proceedings are afforded greater protection from public disclosure in court than top secret national defense information. Hospitals are not completely independent kingdoms. But it would be hard to identify an institution in our society with power over life and death that operates with such broad authority and legal autonomy as the modern hospital.

As a result, any examination of how mistakes are made and corrected in medicine must make the hospital the principal focus. There are other players in the game, including state licensing boards, peer review organizations, county medical societies, and malpractice lawyers. But as the case studies in the next chapters will show, most of the important decisions and actions that affect medical care for heart patients are made at the individual hospital level. The next logical step is to examine medicine's crash record. In the jargon of medicine the issue is called the quality of care.

· · ·

PROFESSIONALS IN THE health care field often debate just what is meant by the quality of care. An even more tortuous discussion often follows about how to measure accurately that ephemeral "quality." Learned discourses on this topic fill books substantially longer than this one. These complexities may be sidestepped by focusing on the simpler idea of mistakes in medicine. For any treatment or act among a representative group of patients, how frequently do mistakes occur? While comprehensive national figures don't exist, the most authoritative scientific journals are surprisingly rich in terrifying and specific detail.

Unless the physician correctly identifies what is wrong, any subsequent treatment is unlikely to help. Using a sample of autopsy records Harvard University professor Lee Goldman concluded that a major diagnosis was missed in one out of five cases. In half those cases a correct diagnosis would have saved the patient's life or prolonged it. The most frequently overlooked ailment was the heart attack. A larger study of thirty-two hospitals in the Southwest produced similar results. The autopsy however, is a perfect illustration of 20/20 hindsight.

Diagnosis is a complex process involving scientific reasoning, experience, and fragmentary evidence. So these studies do not reveal what share of these errors could have been prevented. However, the autopsy remains an important way physicians learn from their mistakes. Both the American Medical Association and Goldman warned about the consequences of the sharp decline in the autopsy rate in American medicine. From a peak of 50 percent in the 1940s the autopsy rate declined to 15 percent in 1985. Goldman attributed the decline in autopsies to physician beliefs that autopsy was a time-consuming chore, to the fact they weren't paid for the work, and to fears of malpractice suits should the autopsy disclose they made an error.

When the specific disease has been identified the next key decision is to select the appropriate treatment, or for hazardous and painful therapies, perhaps an additional diagnostic test. For example, before heart surgery a patient must undergo cardiac catheterization. This procedure is risky enough that it is recommended only in the presence of other evidence of a problem, and after simpler and less dangerous tests have been performed. Rand Corporation researchers convened a panel of nationally known experts to examine a representative sample of 1,677 Medicare patients in three states. The panel concluded that 17 percent of the catheterizations should not have been performed. A similar kind of study was undertaken to examine every pacemaker implanted in Medicare patients in Philadelphia County for a six-month period. A special review panel of experts reviewed 382 cases at thirty hospitals. It concluded that 20 percent of the pacemakers should never have been implanted, and expressed doubts about the need for another 36 percent.

Once a disease is diagnosed and treatment begun the next hazard is iatrogenic illness, mistakes in treatment that kill or injure the patient. Hospital-induced illness has been more frequently debated than studied systematically, but a few well-designed experiments exist. For example, Boston University physician Knight Steel studied 815 consecutive patients admitted to a teaching hospital's eighty-three-bed medical service, and published his results in the *New England Journal of Medicine.* His findings ought to cause consternation even among medical professionals. In all, 36 percent of the patients suffered an iatrogenic illness. That included 9 percent so seriously injured by treatment it imperiled life or produced permanent disability. And in 2 percent treatment "was believed to contribute to the death of a patient." Furthermore, nearly half those so afflicted suffered more than one complication. In one of the medical understatements for which dry scientific journals are noted, Steel concluded, "the risk incurred during hospitalization is not trivial."

What kinds of mistakes in medical treatment create such high rates of injury? The largest single cause in Knight's study were side effects of drugs or combinations of drugs. One reason for adverse drug reactions may be the complicated effects of powerful drugs. A more elementary problem is getting the right drug into the right patient. When Eric B. Larson of the University of Washington in Seattle examined drug orders in a Washington state hospital he found, for example, less than 25 percent of the orders for intravenous drugs contained adequate instructions. A nurse seeking to clarify the instructions would be hindered by the fact that 51 percent of the signatures were illegible. Physicians were instructed to write out the complete generic name, but did so only 57 percent of the time. The rest of the time physicians left pharmacists and nurses to guess at the meaning of cryptic abbreviations such as "chloro" and "tyl."

In the most antiseptic of hospital environments infection will remain a hazard, especially among those whose natural resistance is already lowered by disease. But once again the literature discloses instances of sloppy and careless practices. For example, in a Washington state university hospital Richard K. Albert observed one of the most elementary of all sanitary practices, washing hands. Under the pretense of studying the traffic pattern in an intensive care unit, Albert recorded how frequently physicians, nurses, and other therapists washed their hands before or after patient contact.

"We consider that hand washing is necessary after even minor contact with patients or support equipment, because even the limited contact that occurs with taking the pulse, blood pressure, or oral temperature, or just touching the patient's hand, can result in the transfer of organisms that can be recovered up to two and a half hours later," said Albert.

Further, Albert's intensive care patients were specially vulnerable to infection. All had IV lines inserted, half had urinary catheters, and one out of three had other invasive equipment in place. He found the physicians washed their hands only 28 percent of the time; nurses 43 percent of the time. The most scrupulous were the respiratory therapists, who washed their hands 76 percent of the time. Albert repeated the experiment in a private hospital and the results were even worse in every category. (Since this study, the fear of contacting or spreading AIDS has likely improved hygienic practice among a wide spectrum of health care professionals.)

Accurate record-keeping is an essential precondition for any viable strategy to reduce error rates. Furthermore, record-keeping is a straightforward administrative job and free of the uncertainties of clinical practice. However, hospital performance in basic record-keeping appears no better than the record for errors in diagnosis and treatment.

Medicare claims, for example, affect billions of dollars of the taxpayers' money, and are generated from perhaps the most crucial of all records, the patient chart. To measure how well hospitals were performing, the inspector general of the Medicare program examined a scientific sample of records from 239 hospitals, and reported an error rate of 20.8 percent. About half the errors were made by physicians who picked the wrong diagnosis from the patient chart; the others were coding and other administrative errors made by hospitals' clerical staffs.

A second important record from the hospital world is the death certificate. Beyond the obvious need for accuracy for such a basic record of any society, death certificates play another important role of which physicians are well aware. The accumulated death certificates, more than two million each year, are the principal source documents for analyzing the health status of the entire nation. They are the raw data used to identify the major threats to health, and measure progress against disease. Because of the importance of the document, requirements for filling out a death certificate are set by both state law and federal regulation. A team of pathologists at the National Cancer Institute set out to measure how well physicians and hospitals were doing. To keep things simple they only examined a sample of cases where autopsies had been performed, so the underlying cause of death would be unequivocal. Their conclusion: Improper recording of the underlying cause of death was found in 42 percent of the autopsied cases.

Thus from initial diagnosis to final death certificate these studies suggest an alarming pattern of sloppy performance, with major errors occurring in roughly one out of five cases. An expert might find some point of disagreement with the findings of every one of the examples. For example, legitimate differences of expert opinion may account for some instances of inappropriate treatment. In others, such as with autopsy or hospital-acquired infections, it is difficult to determine exactly what portion of the errors could have been prevented. Yet taken together they comprise a body of evidence of extraordinary weight and consistency. All the studies cited above appeared in reputable scientific and medical journals, and were subject to peer review by other experts in the field. The studies came from many sources, affected every aspect of medical care, and involved hundreds of expert participants. That leads to the next question: What kind of system produces performance such as this?

• • •

AN M.D. WITH a valid license can legally practice almost any medical specialty in almost any city in the land. As long as he treats patients in his own office, a physician has enormous latitude in the drugs and treatments, including therapies discredited by impeccable scientific research, or regarded as outright quackery by colleagues. This broad professional independence is in real life substantially limited by the likelihood that most practicing physicians need to admit some of their patients to a hospital. While insured patients may show up at the door of almost any hospital with the expectation of being treated, physicians face an entirely different situation. It is at the hospital door that outside control and scrutiny of a physician's actions begin. It was in a hospital that the physician was trained and became indoctrinated into the culture of medicine. At the hospital level standards of care are set, errors are detected, qualifications and experience examined. To the extent the practicing physician is accountable to anyone outside court or legal proceedings, he is most likely to have to answer to his colleagues at the local hospital.

From a physician's perspective a hospital structure closely resembles a private country club. To get access to the golf course, or in the physician's case to get access to the hospital, the candidate must first be approved by a membership committee. In both cases the committees inspect the would-be member's qualifications and background. Once admitted to membership, other members' committees control the various activities. A country club might have committees to manage the golf course and the swimming pool. A hospital has equivalent committees for the operating room and the catheterization lab. And faced with a difficult dilemma or a problem, the common response of country clubs and hospitals is to have a members' committee look into the matter. This structure is relatively uniform throughout the country because the organization that accredits hospitals prescribes the committee structure and membership in substantial detail.

The physicians' committees, however, do not enjoy a monopoly of power over the hospital. The rivals for control are the permanent hospital staff that operates and maintains the facility, including janitors, aides, cooks, nurses, and some salaried physicians, called the house staff. Larger hospitals now assign full-time employees to investigate incidents reported by the nursing staff, conduct quality studies, and plan infection control programs. Unlike the democratic committee structure of the physician peers, the hospital management is a formal hierarchy under the direction of the hospital administrator. Further, the hospital chief executive does not answer to the physicians, but to an outside board of trustees in the not-for-profit world, or to corporate management among the for-profits.

The resulting structure is a balance of power and mutual dependence. The hospital depends on the physicians because the physicians are the main source of patients. (A physician often has privileges at several hospitals.) But the doctors also need the hospital to maintain a viable medical practice. It is at the hospital they obtain the use of increasingly expensive medical technology and facilities. Under some circumstances loss of hospital privileges can put a physician out of business. Just how meticulously the balance is respected may be seen in one of the fairly recent innovations in hospital structure, the accreditation requirement that all institutions have a quality assurance program. Mid- and large-sized hospitals hire one or more professionals with the specific job of spotting problems in patient care. These professionals are part of and paid by the hospital administration. But the director of quality assurance at a hospital takes any findings to a quality assurance committee, and that committee is part of the network of physicians' committees.

Other recent pressures on medicine have threatened to tilt the physician/hospital balance. For example, more and more physicians are salaried hospital employees, particularly in the emergency department, the intensive care, and coronary intensive care units. Health maintenance organizations, like any bulk purchasers, independently negotiate high-volume, low-price contracts with hospital administrations, thus taking the power to select a hospital away from physicians. The Medicare system of paying a fixed price for each hospitalization inspired hospitals to take new interest in how long patients stay and why.

Two trends have benefited the power of physicians. A long-term trend towards shorter hospital stays has left the nation with a large surplus bed capacity. And the rapid growth of for-profit hospitals has made the industry even more sensitive to the costs of empty beds. Both motivate hospitals to cater to the physicians who can refer patients.

Thus physicians and hospitals need each other more than ever. And despite an era of rapid change, the unique system for detecting and correcting mistakes in medicine survived largely unchanged. Physician committees still rule the hospital on most medical matters. The doctors do not call it country club government or physicians' committees. In medicine it is called peer review.

The task might be deciding whether a new physician has enough training and experience to perform bypass surgery. It might be trying to find out why so many deaths occurred last month in the coronary care unit. Who will tell Jack that he really shouldn't be performing surgery any longer? A plastic airway that was supposed to be firmly lodged in a patient's trachea was inserted improperly and punctured a lung. The pharmacist complains he can't read the terrible handwriting on the drug orders. Should the cardiac surgeons have one of the operating rooms for their exclusive use, forcing other surgeons into a less convenient schedule? All these problems are likely to be resolved through peer review, a process with a particular set of rules, strengths, and weaknesses.

Peer review is a physicians-only club. The strength of the arrangement is that it guarantees that those making these medical judgments not only have a minimum of knowledge, but are applying it in daily clinical practice. The weaknesses are those shared by many groups of insiders with interlocking interests, and similar income, education, and background. Criticism may be restrained by fears that their turn may come next, by friendship, by the need for referrals, or because they are business partners in practice.

Peer review is also secret. Suppose that an emergency department doctor was reprimanded for improperly inserting an endotracheal tube that punctured a patient's lung, and was instructed to undertake additional training. While state laws vary somewhat this information is normally safeguarded from disclosure to the public, the patient, or his family. Proponents say that the secrecy is essential to guarantee candor and vigorous self-criticism among colleagues. It also means that prospective patients, physicians outside the hospital, and state licensing boards cannot examine the primary machinery for correcting mistakes in medicine to determine whether it is working properly.

Peer review is volunteer work. For all physicians it is an additional unpaid duty and responsibility of medicine. Among those paid as fee-for-service, time spent on peer review reduces the time spent treating patients, and reduces their income. When peer review triggers major conflicts among physicians the process can demand hundreds of hours of volunteer time.

One major door remains open into the otherwise secret proceedings of peer review, and it involves one of the most important delegated responsibilities in medicine: the qualifications of physicians. It is a clumsy and antiquated notion to suggest that, overall, physicians are either "competent" or "incompetent." A physician who is perfectly competent to perform brain surgery is probably incompetent in attending a difficult birth. You wouldn't want your surgeon administering the anesthesia, or the anesthesiologist doing the surgery. The more specialized and demanding the medical task, the finer the distinction between competence and incompetence, between qualified and unqualified. In heart surgery, for example, some cardiac surgeons who had pioneered in valve replacement proved unsuccessful in performing the different and much more delicate bypass operation. But as bypass surgery became the dominant open-heart operation, other cardiac surgeons began to warn that some of their colleagues were doing occasional valve replacements without sufficient experience. Numerous surgeons told me a specially skilled anesthesiologist was essential to successful open-heart surgery. But that means that an anesthesiologist who might be perfectly competent for surgery in the abdominal cavity could kill patients in open-heart surgery. The entire problem of establishing the qualifications of medical specialists has been delegated to individual hospitals. When a physician is granted privileges at a hospital it is only to perform those specific medical tasks for which the peers deem him qualified. Perhaps the single most telling sanction of peer review is to suspend, limit, or revoke a physician's privileges. At that point the decision is no longer confined to the secrecy of the hospital.

Most state licensing laws require official and therefore public notice if a hospital revokes or limits a physician's privileges. One critical question on practically every state's license application for doctors is: "Have privileges ever been denied, suspended or revoked?" Unless the answer to the question is "yes," a state license is often routine if a physician has been licensed in another state. A physician seeking to practice at any hospital can expect to be asked if his privileges have ever been limited, and can expect to do a great deal of explaining if the answer is in the affirmative.

Considered as a piece of problem-solving machinery, peer review is missing many of the checks and safeguards found essential in other areas of society. Conflict resolution ranging from a marriage dispute to management/labor differences has traditionally relied on impartial outsiders. Peer review asks such impartiality from the physicians who must judge friends, colleagues, business partners, and competitors. Opening important processes to public scrutiny confers another fundamental protection. Individuals will seldom commit in public view actions frequently undertaken under the veil of secrecy. And anyone who doubts the system is free to observe its operation firsthand. This is the driving logic behind open courtrooms, public records, securities disclosure regulation, and public hearings. Finally, the most important safety functions in society have been long executed by paid professionals. We would not rely on volunteers to insure the safety of nuclear power plants, yet this is the standard practice in the nation's hospitals.

"I'm not defending the perfection of the system," said James S.

Todd, a surgeon and a senior vice president of the American Medical Association. He was summing up a long conversation about peer review. "It's like democracy. It's a lousy system, but it is better than any of the others."

In the following chapters, case studies of how specific hospitals dealt with major questions about open-heart surgery will address the question of whether a lousy system is good enough.

13

A HEART SURGEON'S
WORST NIGHTMARE

South Bend, Indiana, is a rust belt industrial center that has already endured the worst of its decline and has begun a modest comeback. Downtown a picturesque red brick factory beside the St. Joseph River now houses hotel suites and a fancy restaurant. Once it was used for manufacturing steel lathes, and even earlier, Singer sewing machine cabinets. Not all of South Bend has come back to life. The city is still trying to find productive uses for the sprawling auto assembly plant that has been idle since the last Studebaker rolled off the assembly line in 1963. It is lively in South Bend on fall weekends when thousands pack the town for Notre Dame football games. But mostly South Bend is quiet. It offers street after street of well-kept older homes on comfortable avenues shaded by stately rows of oak, maple, and walnut. Outside of town, fields of corn stretch all the way to the horizons. The Michigan border lies just a few miles north and ninety miles west is Chicago.

In the year 1974 a young physician from New Zealand named Ross Gardner came to town. It had been a long journey in every way. To learn how to pilot a high-performance jet fighter takes fifty-four weeks of intensive training. To master the basics of business management requires two years, and a law degree takes three years. To become a heart surgeon takes ten years or more. The training starts in the classroom and the laboratory learning human anatomy, biochemistry, and mastering the arcane language of medicine. Next comes an apprenticeship on the hospital wards, memorizing, watching, taking patient histories, running medical errands. Only then begins the first learning-by-doing, and the rite of passage of all physicians, the internship. Finally, the development of a future heart surgeon's technical skills commences with a general surgery residency. Once a fully-trained general surgeon, the most determined, promising, and talented win admission to a further residency in thoracic surgery, which includes open heart and other operations on the chest cavity. It was such a test of skill and endurance that Gardner had passed.

He had grown up in a tiny dairy farming town in New Zealand and emigrated to the United States after medical school. No sooner had he completed the two surgical residencies at the University of Iowa than he quickly learned that even a decade of highly-specialized training does not immediately open the door to riches and success. After a year as the junior man in a surgical group in Seattle, Gardner selected South Bend to establish a practice of his own.

For a decade heart surgery had been a much-acclaimed specialty, but practiced mainly at major medical centers, especially those where the surgical techniques and technology had been perfected. So there were Michael DeBakey and Denton Cooley in Houston, Donald B. Effler at the Cleveland Clinic and John W. Kirklin at the University of Alabama at Birmingham. The real boom began as ever-larger numbers of cardiologists learned how to perform angiography, and could themselves map out the obstructions in the coronary arteries, identifying ever-larger numbers of candidates for surgery. Then they would pack their patients off to the Cleveland Clinic or the Texas Heart Institute for the bypass operation. Ross Gardner hoped to offer something new to the cardiologists of South Bend. He would perform the heart surgery right there in town. Gardner seemed to have the right new medical service at the right time.

The choice of hospitals was easy. South Bend has just two major hospitals. St. Joseph's Hospital is located six blocks west of the downtown area. On the opposite bank of the river stands Memorial Hospital, and in 1974 it was the obvious candidate for a heart surgery program. A former X-ray room at Memorial Hospital housed the only cardiac catheterization laboratory in South Bend. And when Gardner arrived just one cardiologist in town knew how to make the X-ray moving pictures of the heart that are the necessary prelude to heart surgery. After a committee of the Memorial Hospital physicians determined that Gardner was qualified to perform heart surgery, he opened for business. Back then, Gardner recalled, "It was pretty primitive." He brought his own heart/lung machine and a perfusionist to operate it. He had to train nurses. He practically lived at the hospital.

In nine months he was joined by a partner. The second newcomer was an old friend and fellow resident at Iowa named John Rubush. Gardner's new colleague was a ruggedly handsome Indiana native, a college football quarterback, and graduate of Indiana University medical school. So while Gardner had finally settled down almost at the opposite end of the earth from his birthplace, for Rubush it was almost coming home again. As coronary bypass surgery grew rapidly in popularity, South Bend's pair of heart surgeons flourished and prospered.

American society can spawn a surprising number of millionaires among those with the right skills in the right place at the right time. It happened among Texas oil speculators who were quick and smart enough to cash in on the rapid escalation of energy prices in the 1970s. It happened in California among the electrical engineers and entrepreneurs who grasped the vast potential of the cheap and easy-to-use silicon chip. And similar magic touched those heart surgeons in a position to benefit from the explosive growth of coronary bypass surgery.

By the early 1980s Gardner and Rubush were doing 300 to 400 open-heart operations a year. Their actual income isn't known. But the usual fees paid heart surgeons suggest they had an excellent chance to become wealthy. For example, a typical fee for the principal surgeon in a bypass operation is $5,000. The assistant surgeon is usually paid 20 percent of the principal surgeon's fee, or $1,000. Thus two surgeons doing the same volume of surgery these two performed might share in gross receipts of one million to three million dollars a year. Gardner and

Rubush might have done better or not as well. But million-dollar annual incomes are common among heart surgeons.

Heart surgery is a study in extremes. It is dangerous. It is dramatic. It is difficult. It is lucrative. It requires extraordinary attention to minute detail. It attracts a certain kind of personality. Gardner describes himself as "pig headed." Rubush so loves the operating room that he'd be pleased to remain there all day, mostly dispensing with the physician and patient contact that constitute the bulk of medical practice for other kinds of doctors. So when Gardner and Rubush began to have trouble, it is not surprising that it turned out to be big trouble indeed.

The problems began, as Rubush remembered it, in 1983. Bypass surgery is a drastic and intrusive procedure performed frequently on persons in ill health and with already damaged hearts. Inevitably some patients will not survive what medical jargon describes as "the insult of surgery." Each time a death occurs in surgery the responsibility for reviewing the case falls on the chief of surgery at the hospital involved. That is what the guidelines for accreditation require, and that is what occurred at Memorial Hospital. The chief of surgery is normally not an awesome power figure among the other physicians who wield the scalpel in the operating room. Using public schools as an analogy, the chief more nearly resembles the president of the PTA than the school principal, and the chief of surgery's job rotates as an extra duty among peers. Furthermore, in 1983 when the first signs of trouble appeared, the chief of surgery was Ross Gardner himself. However, the symptoms of the problem were unambiguous. Patients were dying.

Initially there seemed to be logical explanations for the growing number of deaths, at least from the two surgeons' perspective at the time. The hospital was the same. The surgeons were the same. But the patients were changing. Most notably, they were older.

"If you looked at the early years, the average age was fifty-five or sixty," said Gardner. "You did it basically on healthy people who wanted to get rid of their angina. That's comparatively easy compared to a seventy-eight-year-old with diffuse disease not only in the main coronary arteries. It's like plumbing. If you stick water into a pipe that's also blocked downstream, the flow is not going to go anywhere."

They also believed they were seeing more emergency cases, patients with rapidly deteriorating hearts, others with immediate problems. In a world where the critical scrutiny comes from the surgeons themselves on a case-by-case basis, it is not hard to imagine that this explanation seemed reasonable.

This proved a much less adequate answer when the patient deaths at Memorial Hospital were compared with other institutions. It is possible to rank by mortality rate each of the 494 hospitals in the United States that performed at least thirty bypass operations on Medicare patients in 1984. Among that group Memorial Hospital ranked last. In all, 23 percent of the Medicare patients died after bypass surgery in 1984, according to hospital figures. That is a death rate more than four times higher than the national average and almost ten times higher than leading medical centers performing hundreds of these operations a year. Had these comparisons been available in South Bend, they would likely have triggered an immediate investigation. But such nationwide comparisons as this are extremely rare in medicine. And this ranking had not yet been calculated. But even without such stark comparisons, the problems in heart surgery came to a head in December of 1984. For two years the mortality rate had been creeping upwards. Now so many patients would die in a single month that the surgeons themselves were alarmed.

"They still haunt me," says Gardner. "It's horrible. You wake up nights wondering what you did wrong. It was the first time I ever lost two patients in one week." He still remembers one of the cases vividly, an elderly woman who received internal mammary grafts. Twenty-four hours after heart surgery Gardner had her back in the operating room. The grafts weren't open and supplying blood, and had to be replaced. Her heart was still beating when she left the operating room, but she died soon thereafter.

"I never had a month like that, I know," said Gardner. Next the problem spilled out of the privacy of the operating room, and into the South Bend medical community.

• • •

BY 1984, THE position of chief of surgery had rotated to a general surgeon named Thomas L. Poulin, and he was reviewing the surgical deaths.

"It was obvious that they had a lot of end-stage patients, older patients, poor risks," Poulin said. "Even though it [the mortality rate] was a little high, I thought it was probably not unwarranted." Among fiercely independent peers, it's not clear that Poulin felt he could act anyway.

"It is difficult for me to tell another surgeon in the department that he's not doing a good job," Poulin said. "The quality assurance committee really has to handle that."

However, it was not the quality assurance committee but the cardiologists who took action. They employed a tactic that was simple, effective, and dramatic, but found nowhere in the hospital accreditation manual. It is called starving the surgeons.

For heart surgery Gardner and Rubush were the only game in town. However, in a majority of patients, bypass surgery is an elective procedure performed on persons who, except for periodic chest pains, are otherwise in good health. It was not exactly convenient, but perfectly feasible to pack these patients off to Cleveland or Indianapolis for their bypass operations. In fact, some South Bend cardiologists already were doing that routinely. As the cardiologists began to send their patients elsewhere, the effects could be immediately felt throughout Memorial Hospital.

One of the operating rooms had been reserved for open heart surgery. Now it was frequently empty. It meant idle anesthesiologists. Soon the heart surgery problem commanded the attention of the hospital administration, the medical staff, and Poulin.

"As the cardiologists lost some of their confidence in the surgeons it got to the point where the only cases they referred were those who can't travel," said Poulin. It was time for action.

It appeared that the South Bend medical community hoped to handle this crisis the way medical problems were often disposed of in the good old days: so quietly and subtly that no outsider ever noticed anything. A senior vice president of the American Medical Association, James S. Todd, described such an incident during his years as a practicing surgeon:

"I can remember as little as twenty years ago, seeing in my own hospital the peer review system work terribly effectively, terribly quietly. The tissue committee decided that a particular surgeon just wasn't practicing the way he ought to. It was all done in the corridor. No records kept. Within a very short space of time that surgeon was no longer going to the operating room."

Soon Rubush found himself in what he called a "curbstone consultation" with an influential South Bend cardiologist. They talked casually in the corridor of Memorial Hospital. The cardiologists wanted Gardner out. Rubush could continue to practice, but he would have to work with a new surgeon from outside.

Rubush believed he had a political problem on his hands, a conflict of personalities between the admittedly stubborn Gardner and the cardiologists. He even sought outside advice about how to smooth relationships. But a few days later he got the same message about Gardner from the hospital administration. He was so shocked that he took Henry Olivier, a young heart surgeon who had recently joined their practice, to the hospital offices and asked an official to repeat the ultimatum.

The entrance of the hospital into the problem sent the three surgeons into a huddle to evaluate the situation and plan their future moves.

"I told the other guys I was willing to leave if they wanted me to," said Gardner. His two partners refused.

Rubush said, "We got to thinking about it and I said, 'We can't do this.' He and I were residents together since 1966 at the University of Iowa. It just wasn't right." Further, while the criticism centered on Gardner, the two surgeons' individual mortality rates were similar.

When Rubush carried back the message that there was no deal, the conflict escalated to the medical staff, the committee of physicians with hospital privileges.

Rubush began a series of meetings with individual cardiologists, and appeared before the medical staff. "We presented our statistics and said, 'Let's go through these cases. What could we have done differently?' "

During this time they continued to perform a still sharply reduced schedule of heart surgery but were monitored by other physicians.

The conflict moved into its final phase when the hospital and the medical staff turned to an outside consultant to evaluate the entire heart surgery program. They selected John W. Kirklin of the University of Alabama at Birmingham. It was Kirklin who would provide an authoritative answer to the question that would determine Rubush and Gardner's future: Could the large number of deaths be explained by an unusual group of sick patients—or did it indicate problems in surgery?

Kirklin's reputation in heart surgery is based partly on his achievements in perfecting some of the surgical techniques used in bypass surgery. He is also the author of a major textbook on cardiac surgery. Much of his fame, however, came because of his insistence that heart surgery is a science, not an art.

However, Kirklin never set foot in the operating room in South Bend. Instead he collected all the patient charts for the past two years and took them back to Birmingham, where he shared them with a colleague, Eugene H. Blackstone, professor of heart surgery research. Blackstone offers medicine an unusual combination of skills rarely found in the same person: He is both a physician and an expert in biostatistics. Kirklin and Blackstone have built a massive computer file of hundreds upon hundreds of heart surgery cases at the University of Alabama Medical Center. It permits the comparison of the results of two institutions after adjusting for any identifiable differences in patients, based on the detailed information on patient charts. So the authority of Kirklin's surgical knowledge and skills would be combined with the objectivity of a computer analysis of hundreds of comparable cases. Four months later Kirklin returned to South Bend to make his report to the medical staff of Memorial Hospital.

The gross mortality rate in South Bend was about ten times higher than experienced at the University of Alabama, according to figures from the two institutions. In theory, some of that extraordinary difference might be because of an unusually large number of severely ill patients in South Bend. Neither hospital officials nor Kirklin will discuss the report. However, when Kirklin finished presenting his findings to the medical staff of Memorial Hospital, open-heart surgery was immediately closed down for a reevaluation.

"He [Kirklin] said we're terrible," Gardner recalled. "We could see the handwriting on the wall." The Kirklin report and the surgeons' decision to hang together also ended any possibility that they could survive practicing medicine in South Bend. For the short term, however, the heart surgery program soon reopened for business, and the surgeons continued to operate. But the end was now in sight.

With the benefit of what Ross Gardner called the "see-backward scope," the two surgeons can now identify other things that began to go wrong. One critical change came in the cardioplegia, the fluid that is used to protect the heart from damage during the bypass operation. For years the two had used cold crystalloid cardioplegia, a solution of potassium, water, and salt that is injected into the heart through the aorta and sometimes poured over the surface. Following a nationwide trend in heart surgery, they switched to blood cardioplegia. Although countless other surgeons have used blood cardioplegia successfully, the two South Bend surgeons apparently didn't do as well with it. Somehow, the patients' hearts weren't as well protected. The issue is technical, but can be of crucial importance to survival. The less damage a surgeon causes to the patient's heart, the more likely it is to begin to beat again when the operation is complete.

"We had gone to a different technique of myocardial preservation," says Gardner, "which is basically what I think got us into the problem." The two surgeons also made a second change in surgical technique. It too was in response to current trends in surgery.

For many years most heart surgeons had fashioned bypass grafts entirely from segments of vein harvested from the leg. A well-known heart surgeon, Floyd D. Loop of the Cleveland Clinic, had pioneered a technique that also utilized the two internal mammary arteries. In this procedure the mammary arteries are separated from the chest wall but left connected to the arterial blood supply. The free end of each artery is then joined to a coronary artery to supply blood to the heart. The advantages are believed to be twofold: The mammaries are arteries, not veins. Veins are more rigid, not flexible like arteries. Veins also have one-way valves to prevent backflow, and once in place, veins are more vulnerable to obstructions. Also, the internal mammaries proved unusually resistant to the process that produced lesions in the coronary arteries and vein grafts. In well received and widely read scientific studies, Loop has shown that Cleveland Clinic patients did better with internal mammaries.

In South Bend, using the internal mammaries emerged not only as a question of surgical technique but of medical politics. A heart surgeon's most sensitive relationships are not with patients but with their cardiologists. It is the cardiologist who refers the patients for possible surgery, and who most frequently evaluates the surgeon's work. Based on Loop's reports of better results, cardiologists in many communities, including South Bend, started asking the heart surgeons to do internal mammaries. But not every surgeon was as enthusiastic as Loop, nor could they do them as quickly and skillfully as the pioneer who had invented the technique. This was how Rubush saw it:

"They [the surgeons] are pressured by cardiologists, severely pressured by the cardiologists, to do certain things that are against their better judgment. I think that was why we were doing so darn many internal mammaries."

Rubush and Gardner also learned later that they were completing the surgery more quickly than at other major medical centers. Speed in heart surgery can be a result of confidence, experience, and proficiency. But it can also mean sloppy surgery, or indicate a problem called incomplete revascularization. The success of bypass surgery hinges on increasing the total blood supply to the heart. If the surgeons do not bypass all the important blockages, the surgery may do more harm than good. Incomplete revascularization is one cause of death or early rehospitalization after heart surgery.

Within four months of the Kirklin report Memorial Hospital had recruited two heart surgeons from academic medical centers, Philip A. Faraci from Tufts in Boston and James P. Kelly from Tulane in New Orleans. With a big enough potential caseload to generate an income of a million dollars a year it was not going to be exactly difficult to attract top talent. In Gardner and Rubush's bad year, 1984, the mortality rate among Medicare patients reached 23 percent. After Faraci and Kelly completed their first fifty-three operations on Medicare patients, the death rate was 3.8 percent.

• • •

WHEN TED BECK set out to recruit a heart surgeon for the Trover Clinic in Madisonville, Kentucky, he was hardly a novice in checking out a physician's credentials. Beck is the medical director of a large group practice that includes nearly one hundred physicians. While headquartered in Madisonville, the Trover Clinic has six other locations in rural western Kentucky.

"We pride ourselves a great deal on the quality of care we deliver, compared to Lexington, Kentucky, or Washington, D.C., or wherever you want to compare," said Beck. "So in other words, we're on the up and up.

"We have a recruiting committee that screens applicants, and they go through a formal interview, day to a day-and-a-half on site." And in accordance with their procedures they had lengthy interviews with at least two candidates.

Then came the reference checks.

"We do formal checks. The hospital does formal checks. We have formal references related to training and physician peers. And we pick up the phone for what I would term an informal reference."

And for this particular appointment, Beck handled some of the reference checking himself. From the telephone listings, he called four or five cardiologists blind and asked for their candid assessments of the candidates.

"Let me tell you how I handle it," said Beck. "I tell the individual that I'm referencing, that this is off the record, this is a candid, private conversation, and that's where I leave it. I don't even generate a permanent record.

"If a guy's referring patients to somebody, then he has some knowledge of his work. At least the calls that I made, I got excellent references."

Beck specifically remembered calling cardiologists who had worked with the leading candidate for the clinic job. One cardiologist told Beck that the surgeon had operated on his own father. Another said the mortality rate among his own patients was 2 percent or less.

After the day-long visit, and both formal and informal reference checks the recruitment committee selected a new heart surgeon for the Trover Clinic.

His name was John Rubush.

• • •

"I'm amazed, that's all I am. That's all I can say," said Beck when given a brief summary of the events in South Bend.

Rubush, meanwhile, conceded that he hadn't told anyone at the clinic about his experiences at South Bend.

"I sure as heck didn't mention the Kirklin study. I wasn't going to say, 'Hey, Dr. Kirklin thinks we're terrible.' I could not talk about it again. Could I go into an interview and say 'In 1984 we had horrible statistics'?"

Rubush also said his results were better in Madisonville. "I pay stricter attention to detail. We closely monitor the temperature [of the heart]. My cross clamp and bypass times are longer because I take longer and spend more time at the minutiae."

Thus the final chapter in the crisis in South Bend was an effort to conclude the heart surgery crisis so quietly that not a trace of the problem would be visible to the public, to state licensing boards, or even a veteran physician conducting a scrupulous background check. The physicians and hospital administration also avoided using the machinery of hospital privileges. That violates at least the doctrine recommended by the American Medical Association.

John J. Coury, a Michigan surgeon then serving a term as president of the AMA, was asked how hospitals should handle a case where a surgeon had experienced an excessive number of deaths.

"They should stop his privileges," Coury said. "If he has poor results, if he is having results that are out of line with the average, then his privileges should be suspended until he improves himself, or he should lose his privileges if he can't."

Had the hospital followed Coury's advice it would have been nearly impossible to resolve the problem quietly. Indiana state law requires that hospitals inform the state medical licensing board in writing when a physician's privileges are suspended, abridged, or revoked. If such notice had been given, Rubush could not have automatically transferred his license to practice medicine from Indiana to Kentucky. Not only do state licensing boards ask, but hospitals and other bodies also routinely inquire whether privileges have ever been suspended or revoked.

There was little Gardner and Rubush could do about being squeezed out of practice in South Bend, but had their privileges been abridged they could have mounted a formal challenge. That could have forced the hospital and medical staff to specify charges, and prove them on a case-by-case basis.

In this light it is not hard to understand why no action was taken on privileges. But it also explains why questions of physician competence are so seldom officially reported.

The departure from official custom that seemed to work in South Bend was the decision to bring in an outside expert to review the heart surgery program. They not only got the expertise of an authority in the field, but Kirklin also conducted an objective analysis based on comparison of hundreds of cases. Were such comparisons routine in medicine, rather than used occasionally to resolve special problems, it is likely that the problems in South Bend would never have occurred.

14
CALIFORNIA
CONFRONTATION

Nobody can spot exactly when the trouble started. The first event on record happened soon after a young physician named Bill Bommer joined the medical faculty of the University of California at Davis. He had just finished his training as a cardiologist a few miles away at the Veterans Administration hospital at Martinez. His fellowship was under tutelage of the medical school at Davis. But the hands-on experience, diagnosing and treating the patients with heart problems, was at the VA hospital. He had done well. He was among the talented minority invited to make the great leap from student to teacher, and thus became an assistant professor of cardiology. The promotion triggered one change that proved of unexpected significance. He would switch his practice from VA Martinez to the medical school's main teaching hospital, the university medical center in Sacramento.

One of his jobs was to identify those patients who might be candidates for open-heart surgery. In Sacramento the patients could be operated on right there at the university medical center. This was a change from Martinez where most patients were packed off for surgery to the VA hospital at Palo Alto. Soon after beginning work at the university medical center he had a suitable patient who was duly referred to a faculty surgeon.

That first patient died. Given the difficulty of the operation—the simultaneous replacement of two heart valves—the outcome could not have been completely unexpected. Not only is the operation technically demanding, but also reduced output from the failing valves often has weakened the heart muscle. Nevertheless, the death troubled him.

Bommer's second candidate for surgery had excellent prospects. He was scheduled for an elective coronary bypass operation, which is as close to routine as anything in the demanding discipline of open-heart surgery. Furthermore, the patient's left ventricle, the main pumping chamber, was normal. This patient also died.

The deaths of his first two heart surgery patients shocked Bommer. During his advanced training at Martinez he had sent between fifty and one hundred patients to heart surgery. Every one had lived. As far as Bommer could tell only one thing had changed, and that was the heart surgeons. Junior though he was, Bommer could not tolerate this situation. He would send no more of his patients to surgery at the university medical center. His patients would go to surgeons in whose skills he had confidence.

Word of Bommer's boycott spread slowly among the physicians in the cardiology section at the medical center. Soon a message came from on high, from the chief of the cardiology section, Dean Mason. Would Bommer consider resuming referrals to the medical center surgeons? Would he cooperate and help develop a better heart surgery program at their hospital? Although uncertain of the consequences of his decision, Bommer refused.

"I was willing to accept whatever responsibility that was required," he said later. "The most important thing to me at the time was making sure that the patients that I knew and worked with, that I was sure they were getting the absolute best care."

Later events suggested that Bommer was ordinarily a team player, and not by nature a rebel, a maverick, or a troublemaker. He revealed the details of this seminal incident only when compelled to under subpoena. It just happened that Bommer, seeing the situation with the outsider's eyes, was the first to notice a problem. Later every one of the cardiologists on the Davis faculty would be forced to make a series of agonizing decisions in which patients' lives, professional reputations, and medical careers would be at stake. The problems involved were a long time in developing, and required years to resolve. The two patients died in 1977. The consequences of the events that unfolded can be felt to this day.

• • •

MANY WHO ACHIEVE success in competitive fields have pursued their interests with great personal intensity since an early age. This trait was apparent in a blond-haired youth named Dean T. Mason as he grew up in the Washington, D.C., suburb of Bethesda. He was a government kid, son of a U.S. Forest Service officer who had been assigned to numerous western posts before getting a senior job at the national headquarters. Like many other boys growing up in the 1940s, Dean Mason dreamed of becoming a professional baseball player. Nearly every weekend that the Washington Senators played at home Mason would begin a long journey on foot and public transportation that would take him from his wood-and-brick suburban house all the way downtown to Griffith Stadium. For fifty cents Mason got a ticket for the bleachers. But he had mastered the maze of ramps and walkways so thoroughly that he could thread his way unnoticed to the higher-priced but often empty box seats. He also knew the exact spot to wait where, two hours after the game, he could hand the biggest stars their pictures to autograph when they emerged from the locker room.

By the time Mason was a high school sophomore he was a fledgling baseball star himself, a starting pitcher on the school team. When the academic year ended he joined not one but three different teams in separate leagues. What happened next would surprise no one but a driven high school youth who believes he can accomplish anything. Soon Mason discovered that his pitching arm was getting sore. He ignored the pain. By the end of the summer he had done serious damage, and his arm would never again be quite the same. He would later recount with pride that he had actually played professional baseball, pitching for a minor league team during a college summer vacation from Duke University. But the same summer also proved his arm would never again be healthy enough for a baseball career. Then he turned the same intensity and passion towards becoming a doctor.

His college yearbook photo at Duke reveals a serious young man with a square jaw, blue eyes, and a head of blond hair combed carefully and under control. From his youth to present-day conversations Mason revealed a bent towards absolute judgments, to dividing the world into friends and enemies. A high school essay about the first baseball game he ever pitched described the members of the opposing team as "the enemy batters." And in discussing the conflicts that later tore a medical school apart he often described adversaries as "traitors" and "enemies."

Mason remained at Duke for medical school, and this time a sore pitching arm didn't slow him down. Duke didn't award the traditional letter grades when he became a medical student in 1954. The basic grade was simply "pass," and in each course a handful of the best students would be awarded "high pass." When Mason graduated four years later he had been awarded "high pass" in every single course but two. The standout performers in medical school are often encouraged to pursue a career in academic medicine. Faculty pay is substantially less than what can be earned in a prosperous private practice. But the prestige, the power, the variety of the academic world continue to attract the brightest among physicians. In pursuit of an academic career Mason applied to all the right places for his internship: Harvard, Yale, and Johns Hopkins. He was accepted at his first choice school, Hopkins.

While still at Duke another event set Mason on a specific course within medicine. Duke was one of the nation's leading centers of cardiology, and had one of the early cardiac catheterization laboratories. When Mason first saw what took place in such a laboratory he was utterly fascinated. Until catheterization, cardiology had been a specialty largely confined to guesswork about the ailing heart. In the 1950s the heart was an inaccessible organ which could be diagnosed and treated only indirectly. With a stethoscope the cardiologist could roughly deduce the condition of the valves as he listened to the sounds of the leaflets snapping shut. And with an ECG the pattern of electrical activity gave clues whether the muscle had been damaged, and where. A chest X ray produced a faint shadow of the heart, but didn't have enough detail to identify problems except in a few diseases where the entire shape of the heart was affected. Cardiac catheterization was like opening a window directly on the most complex actions of the heart. It provided X-ray moving pictures showing fine details of the entire pump in full operation. Now a cardiologist could see the valves flop open and snap shut with his own eyes. Mason believed that catheterization would bring a research revolution to cardiology, converting it into a dynamic scientific discipline. And he predicted that it would bring a clinical revolution because it would make possible new surgical techniques to repair defects that could now be clearly and unmistakably identified. He proved to be right on both counts.

At Johns Hopkins, Mason was dazzled to work in the same hospital wards as some of the most famous names in the history of medicine. It was at Hopkins that William Osler, perhaps the most famous clinician in medicine, helped elevate medical education from a simple trade school to a rigorous discipline based on science. Just after the turn of the century a Hopkins graduate, Abraham Flexner, had helped mold all of U.S. medical education on the model of the Baltimore institution. Mason believed he was following in the footsteps of the great figures in medicine, and was working among a group of physicians with an uncompromising commitment to excellence. And that was what he loved about Hopkins.

After completing his training in cardiology Mason was soon at work at one of the best of the early cardiac catheterization laboratories. It was located at a clinic at the National Institutes of Health in Bethesda not far from where Mason had grown up. Mason prospered at NIH, becoming a leading expert on catheterization, and publishing scores of research papers explaining functions of the heart now being revealed through the new technique. In a paper still quoted today he unraveled the mystery of why the drug digitalis increases the output of damaged hearts, but has no measurable effect on healthy ones. Then, in 1967, recruiters from California made Mason an offer he soon accepted.

In the flatlands of the Sacramento River valley the mighty University of California was creating a medical school as part of a new campus in Davis. Mason was offered the tenured position of full professor. He would also be named chief of the cardiology section at the teaching hospital, the university medical center. It was being established at the county hospital in nearby Sacramento. He could recruit two other faculty members, and planned to build a world-famous cardiology section from the ground up. He was thirty-four years old.

• • •

One of the most important clinical functions of Mason's new cardiology section was to identify likely candidates who would benefit from heart surgery. Then cardiologists would transfer these patients to the care of the heart surgeons, who at the new Davis medical school were in the Section of Thoracic Surgery. The section specialized in all operations in the chest cavity, hence the name thoracic or chest surgery. But heart surgery was the principal focus, the exciting surgical frontier, the most difficult and demanding of the thoracic surgical procedures. To head the Section of Thoracic Surgery the University of California recruited a thirty-six-year-old surgeon from Stanford named Edward J. Hurley.

For a young surgeon, having been Stanford-trained was a résumé entry much to be desired. Under the leadership of the pioneering transplant surgeon Norman E. Shumway, Stanford University's heart surgery program had achieved a luminous reputation in medicine. Hurley, an honor student at Stanford's medical school, was invited to remain for his internship, surgical residency, and fellowship in thoracic surgery. As was the tradition at Stanford and elsewhere, the most promising of the residents and fellows would be offered faculty positions. Thus Hurley became first an instructor and later an assistant professor of surgery at Stanford.

A medical faculty member must not only be a skillful physician and teacher, he or she must also publish scientific papers. And during Hurley's Stanford years he was listed with Shumway as coauthor of twenty-five research papers, many on heart transplantation in dogs and human beings. On at least nine papers Hurley was the first listed author, which customarily identifies the person who did most of the work.

As Hurley's seniority increased he became the chief cardiac surgeon at the Palo Alto Veterans Administration Hospital, the second and less prestigious of the two hospitals at which Stanford trained its surgeons. During the Stanford years Hurley developed an interest in a particular kind of heart surgery: correcting defects in infants and children.

In an embryo the heart first begins pumping as little more than a muscular, elongated tube. Over the next eight months the simple tube is enlarged, divides, is folded and transformed into a four-chambered pump connected to a complex maze of tubing. This process is not complete until about six months after birth. In approximately one out of every 125 babies this extraordinary evolution is not successfully completed, but many of these flaws can be corrected surgically.

The thoracic surgery section that Hurley would build at the University of California at Davis would reflect both his interest in pediatric heart surgery, and his long affiliation with Stanford. Not only would many of the faculty members who would later join Hurley be Stanford-trained, but also the entire style of operation would reflect the Stanford mold.

There were obvious similarities when Mason and Hurley began work at the new medical school. Both had been nurtured in the nation's most prestigious medical institutions, and both were now going to find out what kind of future they could build on their own. As they taught students in the temporary wooden buildings, and practiced medicine in a former public hospital, it is unlikely either realized how different they would be a decade later.

By the year 1979 Dean Mason could lay claim to having become one of the most eminent members of the Davis medical faculty. He had just become editor of the *American Heart Journal.* The year before, he had served as president of the American College of Cardiology, the professional association of heart specialists in internal medicine. In the same year his Davis colleagues also gave him the Faculty Research Award, acknowledging his prodigious output of published research. His résumé lists more than 1,000 publications including eighty-four entries for the year 1978, more than many academic physicians achieve in an entire career. (Mason's listed research publications, however, included not only noted scientific studies but also a letter to the local newspaper, and testimony before Congress.) One reason why Mason could maintain such an enormous output of research was that he had garnered hundreds of thousands of dollars in research grants from the National Institutes of Health and the pharmaceutical industry. He'd used this money to expand his cardiology section to thirteen research-oriented physicians. And as he guided this research he became a coauthor of practically all the papers written by members of his growing section.

And in keeping with Mason's growing international reputation, he had also joined the ranks of medical globetrotters. As the year 1979 began he was soon traveling through New Zealand, where in ten days' time he gave that country's annual heart foundation address, and lectured or conducted rounds in Auckland, Wellington, Christchurch, and Dunedin. Then on to Australia where he conducted rounds in Melbourne and Brisbane. He next traveled to Florence, Italy, where he delivered a research paper to an international meeting on heart attacks, and later edited the proceedings of the symposium. He continued on around the world, appearing next at the Philippine Heart Association's Tenth Annual Convention. His primary accomplishment there was to win the convention golf trophy. Later he would make two more trips to Europe, delivering papers in Paris and Brussels. Mason also touched many bases on the domestic medical circuit. He delivered the medical honor society's graduation lecture at Loyola in Chicago, and lectured or taught at the University of South Carolina, the University of Wisconsin, and Tufts.

Mason's responsibilities to teach and remain active in patient care tended to surround a fixed event on the cardiology section schedule. Every afternoon, starting at 2:30 P.M. precisely, he would conduct the cardiology consultation rounds. The first group of patients to be presented would come from the cardiology fellows who had been called to other hospital wards to examine patients suspected of having heart problems. Next to be presented were other unusual cases that had been admitted to the cardiology section's own area of the hospital. His particular interest was congestive heart failure, a condition in which the reduced output of a damaged heart begins to trigger a complex collection of other maladies throughout the human body. He was an expert on the precise combination of drugs needed to coax the maximum output of a damaged heart, and minimize the ill effects of insufficient cardiac output. Mason's daily rounds might only be attended by a handful of the fellows, or the audience might form a conga line of medical students, interns, residents, fellows, visitors, and faculty. However, he was absent enough that other faculty members said Mason was not seen in the hospital for weeks at a time.

Because it would become a controversy later it is worth noting what Mason was not doing in teaching and patient care. Many of the patients on the ward had originally been admitted after being examined in the section's Monday clinic. At the clinic virtually all the cardiology faculty would gather to examine all comers who showed up with potential heart ailments. As the boss Mason supervised the section but didn't participate, didn't admit patients and sign the charts himself. He rarely catheterized patients himself. He supervised catheterizations. He taught the fellows how to perform them. He provided his assessment of the difficult-to-interpret cases at section's regular meetings. But Mason rarely had his own patients.

The surgeon Hurley's career, meanwhile, developed in a different direction, and this too would play an important role in how future events would unfold. While Mason was trying to build a reputation in national and international cardiology, Hurley had become active and visible in Davis medical school faculty matters. Any hospital has a profusion of committees. The medical school had its own separate collection of committees, and on top of that were statewide units for all the University of California campuses. Hurley was a regular and active participant in dozens of committees, frequently serving as chairman. His résumé lists eighty-eight committee memberships. Further, he had developed ties to the major powers that ran the medical school and the hospital. He had known the chief of surgery since they were residents together. He played tennis with the hospital director. He had friends in pediatrics and in the Department of Medicine. So Hurley worked hard for the medical school and was visible and well known. It was a distinct contrast to the more aloof and less approachable Mason, who was popular among the cardiology faculty that he had forged into a close-knit unit, but otherwise directed most of his energy outside the university.

The formal organization of a hospital, medical school, and peer review was not structured to accommodate the two men, Mason and Hurley, who would share responsibility for heart patients recommended for surgical treatment. They were on opposite sides of the great divide in the organization of hospital medicine. Mason was among the specialists in the heart, lungs, kidneys, liver, and other organs who were joined together in the Department of Medicine. The surgeons were grouped separately under the Department of Surgery with sections for the specialized operations such as those on the heart and chest. They had different medical traditions and a separate chain of command. The cardiac surgeons were responsible for their own peer review, examining cases and correcting mistakes, accountable to the chief of surgery. Even if the cardiologists reviewed the treatment of the same patient as the surgeons, they would do so separately and privately.

• • •

THE YOUNG CARDIOLOGIST Bill Bommer had raised the first warning flag. Soon other members of the cardiology section began to ask questions about heart surgery at Davis. By 1978 Dean Mason had developed what he later described in testimony as "a premonition of concern." It is a curious phrase, obviously one chosen after some thought and research. He later explained it meant, "We have a suspicion that there may be a problem, but we are not absolutely certain." Mason's premonition came as the accidental byproduct of research, which was always a priority in the cardiology section.

That year Mason was studying the performance of the only routinely available replacement parts for the heart pump: the valves. One model was constructed of plastic and metal. But others were made from aortic valves of pig hearts, which had first been preserved in formaldehyde and then mounted in special housing. The porcine valves had recently become available in a new kind of housing, and Mason and two other cardiologists launched a small research project to compare all three models in patients at the medical center. As they started to examine a series of recent valve replacement cases they discovered that frequently it was impossible to make the comparison. The patients were dead.

Since the cardiologists were not involved in the surgeons' review of patient deaths, Mason asked one of the members of his section to prepare a brief survey of the recent mortality experience at the medical center. Mason was immediately concerned when he got back the crude box score for each surgeon and major kind of operation. It would take a much more detailed study of many more cases to reach a definitive judgment. But now Mason believed it was possible that they had a problem.

About that same time Mason also heard a complaint from one of his former students who had gone on to establish a cardiology practice in Sacramento. One day the former student confided in his old teacher that he was no longer sending his patients for heart surgery at the university medical center.

While the warning signs were now clear, it looked to Mason as if a fortuitous change was going to make this delicate situation easier to resolve. The medical school had just named a new chairman of the surgery department, a San Francisco surgeon named F. William Blaisdell. Now Mason had available an outsider who would naturally want to examine the performance of the thoracic surgery section that reported to him. So Mason was optimistic that he had the problem on its way to solution.

Blaisdell had not even formally begun work at Davis when Mason called his office at San Francisco General Hospital and asked if they could talk. The two men met in Mason's office in Sacramento. Mason explained his concern about the heart surgeons, and showed him the simple tabulation. Blaisdell told Mason he would look into the situation.

Mason also expressed his concerns less specifically to Hurley himself. The two men were then on remote but cordial terms and met socially from time to time. In a hallway conversation Mason informed Hurley that he had heard that some cardiologists in Sacramento were no longer referring their patients for surgery at the medical center. But he did not tell Hurley that he had checked on the mortality rate, or reveal that he had met with Blaisdell. Soon relations between the thoracic surgery section and cardiology section, which were never close to begin with, began to go sour.

Hurley had two main complaints against the cardiologists. One was a minor bureaucratic problem of the kind that can grow into a major irritant when relations aren't good. For years Hurley had been after the cardiologists to send more promptly the typewritten reports from the catheterization laboratories. When someone was catheterized the cardiologist immediately noted the findings on the patient's chart. Later the physician dictated a longer, more formal report which was then transcribed by the hospital typing pool. For many years Hurley had complained that the surgeons couldn't get the full reports before the patients showed up at the surgical clinic to be examined. It was embarrassing, he said. Hurley wrote memo after memo complaining about the matter. Sometimes the cardiologists *were* tardy in dictating their full reports, but mostly it was a typing pool problem entirely outside the control of the section. So Hurley's complaints weren't taken too seriously.

Hurley also wanted more patients for heart surgery. As early as 1977 Hurley wrote to Mason saying, "It has become quite evident that each year we have had a major reduction in the total number of open-heart procedures performed." If the decline continued, Hurley warned, the surgical residents might not get enough operative experience to qualify for board certification. He added:

"In a more mundane matter, of course, future funding of our sections, salary support and income return to our section for academic growth and development will be further limited if we see this decline continue." The implication was not that they should start dispatching candidates for whom surgery would be of little benefit, but that the cardiologists were paying too much attention to research and not seeing enough patients.

In Hurley's mind at least a third problem helped sour the relationship between the two sections: faculty pay. Under the existing pay formula heart surgeons were paid 10 to 20 percent more than cardiologists of comparable experience. At the time Hurley was also chairman of the university committee that handled faculty pay. One Sunday Mason called Hurley to lobby for higher pay for his cardiologists, closing the conversation with the comment, "Remember, you've got a constituency out there." Hurley came to believe that conversation was both inappropriate and constituted a direct threat that if he didn't support the cardiologists' demand for higher pay, he might have problems. Mason saw it as a section chief trying to get what he could for his people, and as an innocent and inconsequential comment. However, Hurley viewed Mason in an even less favorable light thereafter.

A dispute over medical control of post-operative care had more serious potential implications for the welfare of patients. Success in open heart surgery depends not only on the skill and cooperation of the entire surgical team. What happens in the hours after the operation is equally critical. The heart may lapse into a dangerous irregular rhythm. A patient's survival may depend on how quickly unexpected bleeding in the chest cavity is identified and corrected. Complex mixtures of powerful medication are used, and must be continuously monitored. A heart attack, triggered by the stress of the surgery, is a constant hazard. Some heart surgeons hardly ever see a patient again once the surgery is complete. Others practically live day and night in the surgical intensive care unit. In the Stanford model it was the surgeon, not the cardiologist, who was responsible for post-operative care. The cardiologists were not even welcome in the recovery unit. In the NIH model which Mason had learned, the cardiologists were involved in every aspect of their patient's care, even to the extent of following their progress during surgery. And this led to a continuing clash.

"The cardiac surgeons literally had told their own residents that calling for a consultation with cardiology would lead to immediate dismissal from the program," said Glen Lillington, who was acting chairman of the Department of Medicine during this period.

Throughout the year 1978 the decline in the surgical caseload continued as other cardiologists joined Bill Bommer in sending some of their patients, usually the more complicated cases, elsewhere for surgery. It wasn't until the end of 1978 that Hurley found out. One of Hurley's residents discovered a patient had been whisked out of the hospital on the evening before surgery, and sent to San Francisco for the operation.

"I do not think that it is their [the junior faculty's] prerogative to arbitrarily send the patient elsewhere without senior faculty consultation," Hurley wrote to Mason. When he demanded an explanation Mason finally exploded in anger.

"Ed, I can privately tell you that we would run out of paper and pencil if a memo were generated from us to you over every instance in which we have been greatly displeased. Such an exchange would be counterproductive, and the results disastrous for both our services." And as a threat and an example, Mason listed six specific operations in which he alleged that surgical errors had been committed.

However, just as relations between the two sections began to reach the crisis level, Blaisdell was following up on Mason's complaint and had completed his own look at the heart surgery program. Blaisdell went into the operating room and watched what went on. He had already known Hurley for many years, and had great confidence in his skills. He checked on the references of one of the other cardiac surgeons in the section. "One of the finest pairs of hands I've ever trained," was the report. Thus Blaisdell reached the firm conclusion that nothing was wrong with the heart surgery at the university medical center.

It is also worth noting what Blaisdell did not do. During 1978 he was not reviewing the deaths in heart surgery. He left that job to Hurley and the other heart surgeons in the section. To the extent any review occurred, the deaths were discussed when the heart surgeons met to discuss cases every two weeks. Blaisdell also did not know or calculate the mortality rate for any of the open-heart procedures, so he could not compare the results at the medical center with what surgeons were achieving either at two other hospitals in Sacramento, or at leading university medical centers. Except for one annual report prepared by the chief resident, Hurley did no mortality studies of his own. Both Blaisdell and Hurley attributed the deaths that occurred to high-risk, sicker patients. But neither one had conducted a systematic study of any kind to demonstrate that this was true.

Hurley and Blaisdell blamed the growing tensions between the two sections on a problem of a radically different character. In their minds it was a personality problem, specifically a Dean Mason problem. They came to believe the source of the difficulties was a chief of cardiology with too big an ego, a section that gave too much emphasis to research, and not enough attention to the more mundane job of teaching and patient care.

And thus what should have been a problem-solving effort focused solely on the safety and welfare of the heart surgery patients had hardened into a direct conflict among proud and powerful men. On one side was cardiology, a large and productive section led by one of the medical school's biggest names. Now arrayed in firm opposition were the two surgeons, who made a formidable team: Hurley, the well-known and well-liked heart surgeon who was tireless in his university committee work; Blaisdell, the forceful chairman of an important department. This was the atmosphere in which any mistakes in one of the most demanding and difficult procedures in medicine would have to be identified and corrected.

Having achieved nothing by talking to Blaisdell informally, Mason changed his tactics. To separate the pressing medical questions from the clashes of personality, Mason wanted an impartial third party to review the heart surgery program. It could be either the Quality of Care Committee right there in the hospital, or an outside expert. And to get this accomplished he turned to the formal chain of command at the medical school.

As chief of the cardiology section Mason reported to the chairman of the Department of Medicine. And that was the office to which he first turned for help. He asked the acting chairman, Glen Lillington, to approach Blaisdell about getting a third party to look at the problem. Lillington talked to Blaisdell, but reported back that the chief of surgery was unsympathetic.

The court of last resort was the dean, the only medical school official with authority over both departments. So armed with some additional mortality figures, Mason sought a meeting to review the situation. The chances of a decisive solution probably were not enhanced by the fact that the medical school was then being run temporarily by an acting dean, a psychologist named Morton Levitt.

However, it was not Mason but the forceful and confident Blaisdell who dominated the meeting with the dean. There was no problem in cardiac surgery, he said. Hurley was one of the ten best heart surgeons in the country. And then he added, "Besides, any monkey can do cardiac surgery."

Mason had with him at the meeting his principal deputy, Anthony DeMaria, who snapped, "Then get us one of them."

The dean sided with Blaisdell, agreeing that an outside review wasn't necessary. He urged both sections to work more closely together.

Meanwhile, more members of the cardiology faculty came to Mason asking if they could refer their more difficult cases to other hospitals. "I told them to let your conscience be your guide," Mason said.

• • •

THE CARDIOLOGISTS' EARLIER studies of surgical mortality had been remarkably simple. A medical student or one of the cardiology technicians was sent down the hall to the thoracic surgeons' office where a logbook was kept. It listed all the cases, the surgeons involved, any complications, and whether the patient had lived or died. It was the chief resident's job to keep the logbook posted. For an earlier spot check a medical student had copied out verbatim every word that had been written in the book for the past six months. Then one of the senior cardiologists had prepared a crude tally that filled two pages on a legal pad. As the controversy grew hotter the cardiologists wanted a more complete and accurate picture of how their heart patients had done. It was September 1980 when the cardiologists launched their first systematic study.

First they needed a list of all the cases. So near midnight one September evening a cardiology technician walked down the hall to the cardiac surgeons' offices intending to copy the logbook. He was immediately discovered by a surgical resident. What was he doing there? A research project for cardiology. Had it been cleared with the surgeons? No, not really. It also turned out that the logbook was gone from its customary place, and the cardiologists never saw it again.

This meant the audit had to be created from scratch. Every single operation performed at the hospital over the past two years had to be reviewed, just to identify the open-heart surgery cases. The next task was hunting down hundreds of patient charts from the medical records library, or from whoever might have them. Each patient chart was a massive document, typically from fifty to one hundred pages long. As they were found the charts got stacked up in huge piles on the conference table in the cardiology section offices. Only then did the real work begin.

After they finished caring for patients, working with students, and doing the research projects on which their careers depended, the thirteen members of the cardiology faculty had to read charts for the surgery study. On every evening and every weekend for more than two months the cardiologists gathered in the conference room to distill from the bulky charts the details needed for the audit.

"Everybody participated," recalled Reginald Low, one of the cardiologists who worked on the study. "It was just like something you do if you're on the basketball team. You go to the practice sessions."

Just at the time the study got underway the medical school at Davis got a new dean, an endocrinologist named Hibbard Williams. It was only a matter of weeks before Williams heard about both the conflict and the audit. In mid-October the dean's office sent word to Dean Mason to finish any study the cardiologists were conducting in time for a meeting with him in three weeks time. They were hard pressed to meet the dean's deadline.

And it was not until the last minute that Dean Mason began to tally the results. It is in the nature of such statistical research that there are only the barest of hints how a study will turn out until the final results are tallied. Until then there was a growing pile of one-page data sheets, and a shrinking pile of patient charts. But when Mason saw the totals finally emerge late one Saturday night he was deeply concerned. The overall mortality rate was almost twice as high as they had expected from earlier spot surveys. With a new dean from the outside, and a lengthy and careful study, Mason believed that a problem that had been festering for three long years would finally be resolved. The study had no official title, but Mason called it "the Data of Concern."

Mason, accompanied by a delegation from the cardiology section, met with the dean at 5:00 P.M. in the conference room adjacent to the dean's office on the Davis campus. Mason carried a report and all the supporting data sheets in a large leather briefcase. The chief of the clinical area, Anthony DeMaria, was present along with three other members of the cardiology faculty. Mason wanted to leave no room for doubt about what occurred at the meeting, he wanted his faculty to witness the results of so much extra effort, and he sought to make clear to the dean that his concerns about the heart surgery program were shared by the other members of the section.

Hibbard Williams sat at the end of the long conference table. In the first seat on his right was Mason, sitting where he could place each of the thirteen pages of the summary in front of Williams and explain what the tables meant. Arrayed down the table in the other seats were the cardiologists. Mason began a briefing that lasted over a half hour.

Over the preceding twenty-two months a total of 346 elective open-heart surgery operations had been performed for which records had been located. The cardiologists had excluded emergency cases, such as those in shock, operated on while suffering a heart attack, or as a result of a complication in the catheterization laboratory. (However, all of the excluded emergency patients had died.) In all, 16.7 percent of the patients over a twenty-two-month period had died, or fifty-eight persons.

Among the 288 survivors of open-heart surgery, 40 percent experienced major complications. The most frequent problem was a heart attack experienced during or soon after the operation. The list of complications also included stroke, permanent lung damage, irregular heartbeat, and paralysis of the diaphragm. The cardiologists excluded minor complications such as pneumonia, fever, and temporary kidney malfunction. In all, exactly one half of the patients the cardiologist studied either died or suffered serious adverse effects from heart surgery.

Mason dwelt in particular detail on a table that traced the history of 236 patients sent to surgery during 1980. What made this group of special interest was that almost half of them had been referred to nearby Mercy Hospital for heart surgery. The cardiologists had sent the more difficult cases to Mercy, the patients with severe previous damage to the heart, those with a more complicated pattern of blockages in the coronary arteries. Among 103 patients sent to Mercy for surgery just two died. Among the 133 patients operated on at the university medical center 20 had died.

Comparisons with the published and self-reported results of leading medical centers were even more unfavorable. By the cardiologists' count, for example, the mortality rate for the most frequently performed operation, bypass surgery, had been 17 percent at the medical center. The University of Alabama reported a mortality rate of 1.2 percent, the Texas Heart Institute, 1.9 percent; and both the Cleveland Clinic and Emory claimed a death rate under 1 percent. All this information, Mason told Dean Williams, showed the need for a third party to review the medical center's heart surgery program. Mason wanted either an outside expert or the Quality of Care Committee to examine their findings.

Williams had a lot of questions about the study. As Mason would remember it, Williams was "antagonistic and disbelieving." In particular, Williams questioned the comparison with Mercy because the two groups of patients may not have been similar. He asked whether the data had been shared with the heart surgeons. Williams made no response to the request for an outside evaluation. He told the group he wanted Blaisdell and Hurley to see the report. He concluded the forty-five-minute session by saying he had to go to another meeting. In a move that would later become a point of contention, Mason finished the meeting by offering Williams both a thirteen-page summary and a thick binder of supporting data, the individual data sheets on which findings on each patient appeared. Earlier in that meeting when Williams had questioned one of the totals, Mason pushed the large binder across the conference table, saying "check for yourself." But Williams took just the summary.

Afterwards the cardiologists huddled in the parking lot outside to exchange reactions to the meeting. Mason told the group he was discouraged by the reception they had received. For many of those present the session with Williams was also their first exposure to the final results of the study. It reopened the question of what patients could be ethically sent to surgery at the medical center. "You'll have to let your conscience be your guide," said Mason once again. But then he added, "Given these results I don't see how we can continue to refer any patients to the medical center." The flow of patients to heart surgery, which had been gradually slowing over the past three years, would now come to a complete halt.

• • •

NOW PLACED SQUARELY in the center of the desk of Dean Hibbard Williams was a medical crisis of major proportions. By the cardiologists' count one half the patients sent to heart surgery over nearly two years either died or were seriously injured. The human toll included fifty-eight dead and another 115 patients with serious complications that included irreversible damage to the heart, brain, lungs, or chest. Even if the cardiologists overstated the problem by a factor of 50 percent, the number of lives at stake would make a speedy and effective solution essential. In terms of the sensitive and complicated politics of a medical school it was a bitter dispute between two prestigious and important groups of highly trained specialists who need to work closely together. Instead the two sections were not even on speaking terms. It was also a financial threat because both the hospital and the thoracic surgery section depended heavily on the income from the lucrative business of heart surgery. The crisis also touched the central purpose of the institution, medical education, because the cutoff of patients would soon require that the heart surgery training be shut down, and the residents sent elsewhere. Finally, open-heart surgery was a high-profile symbol of medicine at its best. A program was important to the university's image as a leading medical center.

For nearly a month Williams maintained an official silence, despite frantic and repeated phone calls from Mason seeking an appointment. One reason for the delay was that Ed Hurley had departed for a four-week trip to Kuwait as a visiting professor of surgery, and Williams wanted to hear the surgeon's response. It also gave Williams a month to think about the problem and explore the possible solutions. Immediately after Hurley returned Williams made his move. He summoned Hurley and Mason to his office. After the November meeting Mason had become wary, and wanted to bring his deputy, Anthony DeMaria. Come alone, Mason was told.

The dean began with his analysis of the situation: While the cardiologists had concluded that the mortality and complications were unacceptable, it was not possible to identify the precise factors that had caused the problem. In short, it was not clear who was to blame. Furthermore, he criticized the cardiologists for not taking up the audit with the heart surgeons before bringing it to him. He condemned the cardiologists for doing a poor job of sharing the responsibility for the post-operative care of the heart surgery patients. There would be no outside review. Nor would the problem be referred to the Quality of Care Committee. The problem would be solved, and it would be solved quickly, quietly, and without outsiders. Hurley and Mason had six months to identify and solve whatever problems might exist. If they failed to produce significant progress, he would fire them both.*

As Mason left Williams's office he turned to the dean and said, "It appears that when one brings a problem to you, he is the one who is penalized."

"That's right," Williams said.

Williams's orders left Mason in a bind. Mason had prospered in the

---

*Williams had the power to dismiss them from their hospital positions as section chiefs, but had no authority over their tenured faculty appointments.

formal structure of the medical system, working patiently in the chain of command to achieve the textbook solutions. And now, perhaps for the first time, the system had unequivocally failed. A person who was not such a literal believer in following the rules might have seen more alternatives to a position that Mason believed was utterly impossible. He could not possibly work out the problems in heart surgery with the man who, in Mason's view, was at the center of the problem. And he was totally convinced that any competent outside reviewer would agree. But Williams had denied his request for an impartial review of his "Data of Concern." He was trapped. His first reaction was simple disbelief that this could in fact be the case. He immediately asked for another meeting to request reconsideration of Williams's plan.

Mason couldn't get in to see Williams, but a week later Williams's deputy, Ernest Gold, agreed to meet with Mason and two other senior members of the cardiology section. "You can't solve the problem with the problem," Mason said. Gold, however, insisted they give the dean's plan a try. Send some patients to heart surgery, and try to make things work. But the cardiologists were equally adamant. Human lives were at stake. "This is not a dog lab," one of the cardiologists told Gold, referring to the fact that heart surgeons practice surgical techniques on dogs. The cardiologists demanded that Gold outline the arrangements in writing.

Hurley and Mason met several times but nothing much happened. The two agreed to conduct joint conferences to review heart surgery cases, but such meetings were pointless unless the cardiologists referred patients once again. Hurley wanted Mason to provide backup material for his Data of Concern, but Mason refused. "You show me your data and I'll show you mine," Mason said. After some soul-searching, and in an effort to follow Williams's directive, fourteen patients were sent to the heart surgeons. No deaths occurred, but when several experienced complications, no more patients were referred.

Through a fluke Mason almost got a review by the Quality of Care Committee. At the December meeting a hospital officer asked who was going to pay for the ambulances being used to transfer heart patients to Mercy Hospital. In the ensuing discussion the Quality of Care Committee learned for the first time that the cardiology section would not send their patients to surgery at the medical center. Mason was invited to attend the January meeting to explain. However, Gold, the deputy to Dean Williams, told Mason not to attend. Mason sent the chairman a note saying he was unfortunately not available.

One evening in January Mason returned to his hospital office to discover that his office had been searched, and various files and records were now missing. The financial books and records of the cardiology section had been seized. Cardiology, one of eleven sections in the Department of Medicine, was the only section with the authority to keep its own books. The section's financial independence had developed because it had received such a large volume of research funding from the outside. (Its patient care income was also double that of any other section.) The seizure, Mason learned, was ordered by the new acting chairman of the department, a hematologist named Jerry P. Lewis. The section's financial independence had been revoked, Lewis told Mason, to resolve questions about fund account balances.

Just two weeks later Hurley and Mason were summoned to the dean's office to report on the progress they had made resolving the heart surgery problem. Williams asked if Mason was ready to resume referring all section patients for surgery at the medical center. Mason said he was not. Had the two men made significant progress in resolving their differences? Hurley indicated a few positive steps had been taken, but added that he still didn't have patient names and the other particulars from the cardiology audit. Mason told Williams he did not think any progress had been made.

It looked like only another stalemate. Later that day Edward J. Hurley resigned as chief of the thoracic surgery section, but would remain as a full professor and active heart surgeon. He cited his inability to get the support of the cardiology section as the reason for quitting. Mason would also be out of a job, but his departure would not be nearly so tidy.

A memo from Blaisdell, still head of the Department of Surgery, hinted that more trouble lay ahead for Mason. Just a few days after Hurley's resignation, Blaisdell urged that a committee begin seeking a successor immediately. He said, "Moreover, the same brush which has tarred thoracic surgery will be turned on cardiology. A fundamental weakness is we have no clinicians of stature in this field who are primarily committed to clinical care."

The next month Dean Mason was asked to resign. The word came from Jerry P. Lewis, who was Mason's immediate superior as acting chairman of the Department of Medicine. But in a telephone conversation Lewis did even not mention the cardiac surgery controversy. Instead he focused on the section financial accounts, which he said were out of balance. An angry Mason refused to quit. "Everything you are undertaking is harassment and a frame-up and you know it," Mason said.

Next came an unlikely development that can only happen in academic medicine where the participants have global commitments. The crisis was placed on hold because the participants left town. In December when Hurley faced a deadly serious challenge to his medical career he left for an extended trip to Kuwait. Now Mason faced a demand for his resignation and promptly departed for a three-week, State Department–sponsored trip to China. Lewis, who wanted Mason replaced, waited for several weeks, in part because of his own travel schedule.

While Mason was still in China, Lewis named Mason's principal deputy, Anthony DeMaria, as the new chief of cardiology. Although Lewis announced the appointment in a memorandum, he apparently did not check first with DeMaria, who refused to take the job. (A few months later he would accept an equivalent position at the University of Kentucky at Lexington, telling colleagues he wanted to leave "this crazy place.") A chagrined Lewis later told the section, "I . . . am sorry that some uncertainty has arisen as I pursued the identification of a new division chief." And then the next day he unequivocally fired Mason.

"Dean, I really consider this to be very serious," Lewis wrote. "You have been removed as the Chief of the Division of Cardiovascular Medicine. . . . You can view this as your having been fired from the position." The audit of the surgeons is nowhere mentioned in this curious letter which included statements such as: "You are rarely in your office. . . . You have not handled promotion matters and merit increases well. . . . There has not been any attempt to balance [the books]."

However, another reason for Mason's dismissal soon emerged. Seeking to stabilize the situation, Lewis met separately with each member of the cardiology faculty. When one of the cardiologists told Lewis the section wanted Mason restored to his position, Lewis replied:

"I have it from Dr. Williams that Dr. Mason will never be Chief of Cardiology again so long as he is dean of the School of Medicine." With Mason removed, it also appeared that cardiac surgery would soon resume. Hurley scheduled three pediatric cases. One of the other surgeons lobbied the cardiologists, telling them it was time to start referring patients for surgery. Heart surgery would likely have resumed at the university medical center had it not been for a woman named Diane Divoky.

15
THE SEARCH FOR
A SOLUTION

Diane Divoky was an experienced newspaper reporter, but she was the new kid on the block when it came to medicine. The Cleveland-born Divoky spent years covering education, and got the medical beat at the *Sacramento Bee* just about the time the cardiologists finished the audit of heart surgery. Armed with a *Physician's Desk Reference* and the *Merck Manual,* she labored to make sense of the complicated technical world of medicine. She also had to face competition from the other newspaper in town, the *Sacramento Union.* Her opposite number at the *Union,* Jeannie Esajian, had covered medicine much longer and had better contacts in the Sacramento medical community. During the first week in June 1981 Divoky was particularly worried about the competition. There was a rumor that Esajian had a big story about the medical center, and it could break at any time. Divoky was frantically trying to get a piece of the story first, whatever it was. Finally, on Friday, June 3, she got the barest of hints from a former resident at the hospital. Find out why the cardiologists send their patients to other institutions for surgery, he said.

The problem was Divoky didn't know any cardiologists. So how could she get some stranger to spill a story that important when she didn't even have a single name? Then she remembered a recent article in *Time* magazine. It had quoted someone at the medical school. His name was

Garrett Lee. So she called and asked for an interview, deliberately omitting the subject she wanted to talk about. Lee liked to give interviews about advances in cardiology, and agreed to talk to her. But he had no time available until Sunday evening. He could meet her in the basement of the medical center, in the echo cardiography lab.

This was not what Divoky wanted to hear. She had a date Sunday night, and she didn't want to cancel it. But since it was notoriously hard to get physicians for interviews she decided to do both. That Sunday evening she told her date she had to stop off for an hour to see someone. Then she would be back. She searched out Lee in the basement. Lee is a boyish-faced man of Oriental extraction whose face radiates energy and animation. Despite his youthful looks, he had one of the most important jobs in the cardiology section: head of the catheterization lab. Divoky's heart sank as she saw not one, but two people in the small basement office. "He's got his supervisor there. I'll never get anything." She was wrong.

It wasn't Lee's supervisor, it was a colleague who left when he saw that Lee had company. Lee had expected that Divoky wanted to talk about balloon angioplasty, which was then a new therapy. Instead she asked, "Why are you sending your patients to other hospitals for surgery when you have a fully certified program right here?" And in that instant the entire course of the controversy was unalterably changed because Garrett Lee decided to tell her the truth.

It happened almost without thinking, but he explained later why he suddenly spilled out the whole story:

"No one was paying attention to the long hours of hard work, that we've being trying to tell the university to improve the quality of care, to get their house in order.

"Cardiovascular surgery was still going on, and the surgeons were seeking out patients for surgery, and the data was essentially covered up."

So Lee told her about the audit and the problems with heart surgery, and he told her that Dean Mason had been removed. What Divoky really wanted was a copy of the audit itself. But Lee didn't have one immediately available, and Divoky's date was soon going to be outside in the car. So Lee said she could have the audit Monday morning. He would leave it for her at the information desk. It is likely that neither

Divoky nor Lee imagined the dimensions of the controversy that would be triggered.

Monday morning Divoky sent a messenger to the hospital and soon had the report in hand. Now she still needed comment and confirmation. She reached Blaisdell, the chief of surgery. He confirmed one fact. There wasn't much heart surgery going on at the medical center. But Blaisdell didn't hint at any problem. He told her they were allowing other hospitals to perform the routine heart surgery while preparing to do pioneering and experimental heart surgery appropriate to a center of their stature. When Divoky asked what kind of experimental heart surgery Blaisdell did not elaborate.

Divoky interviewed Jerry P. Lewis, who had fired Mason. He told her that the quality control process at the medical center was the finest found in any hospital anywhere, guaranteeing superior medical practice.

She also reached Hibbard Williams, and asked what was going on. Williams gave her still another explanation. The fall-off in heart surgery, he said, was because Hurley had resigned. Thus the change in administration was responsible for a temporary decline in the heart surgery caseload.

Hurley was straightforward. He told her he had resigned because of problems communicating with Mason. The 1980 mortality rate, he said, was 12 percent, a result that was "not outstanding, but reasonable given the patient population we saw."

Divoky also reached Dean Mason. He confirmed that the document she had was in fact the audit, and he called the results "catastrophic." Because Mason was the only cardiologist quoted in the resulting story university officials would blame Mason for leaking the story for many years thereafter. When the *Sacramento Bee* appeared with the story it would have an explosive effect. Heart surgery was just beginning to come back to life at the medical center. But as soon as the *Bee* hit the streets, heart surgery at the medical center was finished. Resuming it would become the least of the center's problems.

• • •

WHEN HEART SURGEON Edward J. Hurley saw the *Sacramento Bee* his first thought was the three pediatric cases he had scheduled. He telephoned Tom Riemenschneider, the physician who had referred the patients, and told him to call the families and cancel the operations. Sacramento is the state capital, and the story also came to the attention of Barry Dorfman, then assistant director of the Department of Health Services. The department licenses hospitals. Dorfman told his staff, "I think we have to assume we have received a complaint." A team of investigators was dispatched to the hospital. Physicians in California are licensed to practice medicine by the Bureau of Medical Quality Assurance, which is called BMQA and pronounced "Bum-Qua." Investigator David Thornton would soon begin an inquiry into the competence of the cardiac surgeons at the medical center. The news reports also came to the attention of officials of the Joint Commission on the Accreditation of Hospitals in Chicago.* The Joint Commission quickly realized that the routine survey that had been previously scheduled would not now be sufficient for a hospital whose performance was under fire. The commission assembled a special team to fly to California.

In the Sacramento legal community Divoky's story was also read with great interest. Medical malpractice is difficult to prove in court, particularly in heart surgery, where death is not an unusual outcome of treatment. But the story had one striking passage, that in legal terms was a kind of smoking gun. The audit alleged that similar patients were less likely to die at three other local hospitals. To the trained ear of a malpractice attorney these were critical words because a lawyer must prove not only that a patient was injured or killed, but also that the care provided was lower than the standard of care in that community. That, in so many words, was what the audit seemed to assert. If that conclusion could be proven, it would support dozens of malpractice actions.

Dean Mason read the story with a mixture of relief and anxiety. Finally something would be done, he believed. For Dean Hibbard Williams a difficult problem he had tried to solve in secret with just two people, Mason and Hurley, was now going to involve the full glare of public scrutiny and a cast of hundreds.

---

*The organization is now called the Joint Commission on the Accreditation of Healthcare Organizations.

Thus it happened that newspaper and television reporters, state investigators, the Joint Commission accreditation team, and the BMQA staff descended on the hospital like a horde of locusts. As they did, the medical school administration had to face one particularly difficult and potentially embarrassing problem. The officials were in an extremely poor position to debate the merits of the cardiologists' audit because they had nothing except thirteen pages of summary tables that Mason had presented nine months earlier. There had been no internal evaluation of heart surgery. No outside study. No request for additional data. So little had been done that no one could even say for sure which cases the cardiologists had included in their survey.

It was altogether possible that Diane Divoky, BMQA, and state investigators might have learned from the cardiologists specifics about which the school administration was still entirely ignorant. Not only were they going to have a difficult time explaining why so little had been done about an important allegation involving patients' lives, they could not even produce a copy of the survey and its supporting data. Thus getting a complete copy, especially the data sheets on individual patients, became an urgent priority.

The first request was low key. James Foerster, Mason's successor as chief of cardiology, asked him for a copy of the backup data, explaining he needed it for a strategy session with university lawyers to figure out what to tell state investigators. Mason did not respond. Next the Quality of Care Committee sent Mason a certified letter requesting the full study. Once again Mason did not immediately reply. The next level above the committee was the medical center chief of staff, who was less polite, and formally demanded a complete copy. Mason still didn't deliver one, writing back that he would respond after getting proper legal advice. Finally the conflict escalated to the highest authority at Davis, the office of the chancellor. Executive Vice-Chancellor Elmer W. Learn insisted that Dean Mason produce the audit and the supporting data at a meeting with himself, Dean Williams, the executive director of the hospital, and the chief of the medical staff. One can only speculate how events might have developed differently if the senior university officials had paid this kind of attention to the audit nine months earlier.

However, the sudden and intense interest in the cardiologists' audit did not exactly put Dean Mason in the driver's seat. The survey was a serious and systematic review by experts in the subject, but they'd worked in a rush, barely finishing before the meeting with Williams. The cardiologists knew they had missed some cases. Although it was a section known for its prolific publications, the audit clearly did not meet standards for a medical journal study. Later the cardiologists would say it was never intended for publication, specially in a newspaper, but only to spur the university into getting a third party to perform a systematic review. Nevertheless it was clear that the quality of the audit was going to be on trial just as much as the quality of the heart surgery. So as the university was frantically trying to get a copy, Mason was revising and fine-tuning the details of the audit.

Finally the day arrived when Mason was going to hand over the complete and now revised study. But first Mason and Bill Bommer drove downtown to give a copy to the state investigators, who had joined the crowd of those eager for the document by issuing a subpoena for it. The next stop was the chancellor's office, fifteen minutes down the interstate in Davis. Mason and Bommer were to meet in the parking lot beside the chancellor's office at 3:00 P.M. But when Dean Mason arrived, Bommer, who had the data, was mysteriously missing. Mason stood around the parking lot getting more and more nervous about what had happened. Then suddenly a police car roared into the parking lot. Mason knew the survey he had been under such pressure to produce was something of a medical bombshell, but he didn't anticipate police involvement. In this instance his worst fears were not realized. Bommer's car had broken down on the interstate, and he had flagged a police car so he wouldn't be late. Mason and Bommer gave the material to the executive vice chancellor, Elmer Learn. He handled the large sealed package tenderly, almost as if it were indeed a bomb.

· · ·

IT WAS NOT until nine months after the survey had been submitted that an official body of the University of California first met to consider the merits of the cardiologists' allegations about open-heart surgery with members of both sections present. It was September 1981, and what transpired was no less remarkable than the other events in the controversy.

The meeting was convened by Joe Tupin, a psychiatrist who was acting in his capacity as vice-chairman of the Quality of Care Committee. Edward J. Hurley and the other two cardiac surgeons, Todd Grehl and Robert L. Treasure, were present. But just four of eleven cardiologists were invited. Tupin immediately gave the floor not to the cardiologists to outline their concerns, but to the cardiac surgeons. Hurley went first to describe the controversy from his point of view.

The problems between heart surgery and cardiology, Hurley said, were caused by a lack of communication between himself and Dean Mason, and this clash had led to the audit. Hurley had been unable to respond to the audit for many months because Dean Mason wouldn't provide the supporting data for his survey. Hurley described the cardiologists' audit as the "Dean Mason statistics," and said they were "erroneous and incomplete." The cardiologists had failed to review more than one hundred patient charts. Furthermore, they had counted as dead two patients who were, in fact, alive. The cardiologists had also classified as "elective," patients who in fact were at "high risk." The large number of these high-risk patients made it wrong to compare the medical center's results to other institutions.

As Hurley began a case-by-case review of each of his deaths, one of the cardiologists, Ezra Amsterdam, interrupted. The surgeons had had months to prepare this explanation, but the cardiologists first learned about this session two days earlier. It doesn't really matter what the surgeons think, he added, or even what the cardiologists think. This is a pointless exercise without an impartial third party to examine the problem.

Hurley answered that the surgeons wanted to provide their point of view, and continued with his cases. After the other two cardiac surgeons presented their cases, Tupin called on Peter Doyle, a Sacramento lawyer who was taking a lead role in defending the university against the malpractice suits filed after the disclosure of the audit.

Doyle said he was concerned that both the cardiologists' reputation and their bank accounts might be at stake. The public didn't know the difference between a cardiologist and a cardiac surgeon, and so they also would be blamed for the problems in heart surgery. Furthermore the cardiologists would have to pay any punitive damages out of their own pockets because the university's malpractice insurance did not cover such judgments. The cardiologists could also face legal action for libel and slander for providing the information to the newspapers. The two groups "should not lock horns," Doyle said, and should work together "to defeat the Dean Mason survey."

The four cardiologists were concerned about the tone of the session, and asked for an immediate meeting that would include all eleven members of the section. Later that day Tupin and Peter Doyle held a second meeting with the entire section except for Dean Mason, whom they excluded. Peter Doyle spoke at length.

The public release of the audit data had caused extraordinary problems, Doyle said. The problems included billions of dollars in lawsuits. Reduced income for the medical center. Potential loss of hospital accreditation. A danger of losing the hospital's license. The surgeons faced possible loss of their licenses to practice medicine, and had suffered irreparable emotional, personal, and professional harm, he said.

Why, one of the cardiologists asked, was Mason being excluded from this meeting? The surgeons refused to meet with Mason, Tupin said, and were concerned that he would leak their data to the press. Doyle added that a slander suit against Mason was a possibility. He also wanted to protect Mason from making slanderous statements.

Some of this animosity had been aggravated by a quotation attributed to Mason in a publication called *Medical World News*. Its San Francisco-based correspondent, Judy Ismach, had interviewed Mason at length about the audit. She asked if the real problem was primarily a clash of personalities. Mason's response would be indelibly etched in the surgeons' minds thereafter. Her story concluded with this quote:

"It's true we have personality differences," says Dr. Mason, "but that's not the issue. It's why surgeons are killing people."*

---

*Almost a full year later Mason would deny making the statement, and seek a retraction. *Medical World News* insisted the quote was accurate, and refused to make a correction.

• • •

THE IMMEDIATE CONSEQUENCES to the medical center were ultimately not quite as severe as Doyle had foreseen, but were nevertheless substantial. The state Department of Health Services was the first to move against the medical center. It identified sixty-six deficiencies, and demanded that the hospital submit a plan of correction, or risk losing its license. The state investigators did not examine the results of the heart surgery program specifically, but instead focused on the peer review process.

"What I encountered when I looked at cardiac surgery was a lack of peer review across the board," said Barry Dorfman, the state official who headed the investigation. "It was inadequate when you looked at cardiac surgery, but it was also inadequate when you looked at the other services. In one instance they let the person who was under review supply the data."

The state survey also alleged that the Quality of Care Committee did not hold regular meetings, and noted that neither that committee nor the medical staff examined the problems identified in cardiac surgery. "There was no evidence that the surgical performance of the thoracic surgeons was ever reviewed," the report said.

While the State of California repeatedly rejected the university medical center's proposals for correcting the deficiencies, its hospital license was never revoked. Approximately nine months later the state accepted a plan for improving the hospital, including a moratorium on heart surgery. Later the hospital was placed on four years' probation.

The Joint Commission on Accreditation of Hospitals, after months of assessment and internal debate, revoked the university medical center's accreditation. It marked the first time it had taken such action against a hospital operated by a medical school. The Joint Commission also did not examine the heart surgery program, but the principal deficiencies it cited involved ineffective quality assurance, the same problem that Dorfman identified.

The university medical center, however, avoided having to close its doors by appealing the Joint Commission's revocation. In the additional year it took to lose the appeal the university had made enough progress to win a new accreditation.*

After a lengthy investigation the state Bureau of Medical Quality Assurance took no action against the heart surgeons' licenses to practice medicine. A news report in the *Sacramento Union* alleged that BMQA had found "merit" in allegations, but insufficient evidence to prosecute. However, BMQA releases such findings of "merit" only to the physicians involved. When asked later Hurley said he could not recall what BMQA had said.

The wave of outside investigation left the university medical center battered, but barely touched the central issue that triggered the entire episode: What had happened in heart surgery? Had anything gone wrong, and if so, what? It was the surgeons themselves who seemed to provide the opportunity to address that pivotal question specifically, fairly, and in public. Hurley and the other two surgeons sued eleven members of the cardiology section and their employer, the university, for libel and slander.

First they charged that the audit of the heart surgery program was false, misleading, and inaccurate. The cardiologists failed to evaluate 127 patient charts, and had not included eleven patients whose files could not be located. The audit reported two patients as dead who were in fact alive, and counted one patient twice as having complications. Some operations were attributed to the wrong surgeon.

The second major issue ran directly to the core of the controversy, and focused directly on the issue that all the other inquiries and investigations had avoided. The surgeons denied that the death rate was excessive, and claimed their results were similar to other medical centers. The surgeons' suit said:

"The statistical mortality and morbidity rates of surgery performed by plaintiffs compare favorably with those of other thoracic surgery programs of like kind, having similar patient bases, and like criteria for surgery."

---

*Accreditation is not required by law, but in California the hospital could not get paid for treating Medicaid patients unless it was accredited. With the second largest volume of Medicaid patients in the state, the hospital would have been quickly forced out of business.

As the cardiologists reviewed the suit with their university-appointed lawyer, Claude A. Smart, they told him they wouldn't pay the surgeons a dime. Mason, still smarting from his removal as chief of cardiology, welcomed the suits as an opportunity to vindicate himself in open court. The cardiologists believed they had convincing answers for several of the allegations about factual errors. For example, it was true that they had not reviewed 127 raw patient charts; they had accepted the information on those patients contained in the surgeon's own records. Furthermore, even if every one of the procedural allegations were true, it would have little effect on the key question: the overall mortality rate.

Therefore the death rate was the critical issue that both sides would have to address in open court. The surgeons swore that their results compared favorably with similar programs treating similar patients. The cardiologists alleged that the surgeons experienced more patient deaths even when referred only the simpler and more straightforward cases.

When the surgeons' lawsuits were dismissed two years later, the cardiologists believed they had been vindicated at last. Although the case had never gone to trial, they had not paid a penny in damages, apologized, or backed away from their position. But their university-appointed lawyers had not told them the full story about how the lawsuit had ended. The University of California, which was also a defendant, agreed to pay the surgeons two and a half million dollars in damages.

The smallest award went to Robert L. Treasure, who had operated at the medical center for approximately one year before the heart surgery program was shut down. Treasure received $150,000 in cash and $20,000 a year for the rest of his life.

The largest cash payment went to Todd Grehl, the surgeon shown with the highest mortality rate in the cardiologists' audit. Grehl would receive $490,000 in cash. He would also get monthly payments for the rest of his life. They would began at $40,000 annually and increase to $60,000 a year.

It was Hurley, however, who was most fully protected in the settlement. He received $275,000 in cash and $20,000 annually for the rest of his life. He also was guaranteed an administrative job at the medical school at his current salary of $116,344. Furthermore he was promised that he would not have to work at the new job for at least two years, receiving one year as a sabbatical, and a second as leave with pay. Finally, if heart surgery was reinstituted at the university medical center, Blaisdell would support Hurley as a participant. Notes of the meetings held to arrange the settlement showed it was Blaisdell who promoted the awards, especially to Hurley. There was one important stipulation: The $2.5 million in payments had to remain secret. Dean Mason, meanwhile, was driven out of the medical school at Davis.

• • •

HE ASKED HIS wife Maureen to come along. Dean Mason was normally a man who tried to keep his work and his family life separate, but this was different. Later he said he invited her so she could witness the occasion herself, and he would not have to talk about it again. They went to the office of his lawyer, Frank Iwama. It was the morning of September 28, 1982, almost two years after he had handed the audit of the heart surgery program to Dean Hibbard Williams.

First Mason had lost control over his section's finances. Then he was removed from his job as section chief. Next the university tried to revoke his hospital privileges, which would end his usefulness at Davis as a physician. While he was battling to retain his privileges he was not actively treating patients. Therefore his salary was cut in half. To make the message extremely clear, all the furniture had been removed from his office at the hospital.

They met in Iwama's conference room and were soon joined by John F. Lundberg, one of the medical school's lawyers. Enough time had passed so that the atmosphere was restored to civility. Lundberg had with him a group of documents. One letter was from Dean Hibbard Williams.

"I have found no evidence to indicate that your handling of the extramural account funds on behalf the division of cardiology involved any personal impropriety on your part," the letter said. "On the basis of such review I am therefore restoring your status as Chief of the Division of Cardiovascular Medicine." Earlier the university had also conceded that he was not accused of "administrative incompetence." Another letter confirmed that his hospital privileges were current.

Lundberg also presented Mason with a check for $165,000. The payment was "full and complete compensation and satisfaction for [any] such personal embarrassment, mental and physical strain, and injury to health and personal reputation in the community."

In return Mason signed a letter of resignation from the hospital staff and the university faculty. In Mason's eyes the settlement was no victory. Many of the other members of the cardiology section had also resigned or would soon leave. It was the final destruction of a cardiology section he had invested fourteen years in building. And the episode was not quite over.

• • •

THE LAST CHAPTERS unfolded in court in Sacramento. Months earlier one of the university's attorneys, Peter Doyle, had said that if they could win the first one or two malpractice suits, the others would be scared off. Thus millions upon millions of dollars were at stake when Kevin White's case came to trial.

Kevin White was the infant son of a bank executive and a high school teacher, David and Janice White. He was just two and a half months old when he was sent to the university medical center for heart surgery. Kevin had been born with narrowing in the aorta that constricted the normal flow of blood and placed the heart under great strain. He was lying on a trolley near the operating room when a passing physician noticed his distress and immediately tried to resuscitate him. But Kevin White had already suffered irreversible brain damage that left him a spastic quadriplegic.

The Whites' attorney, Morton Friedman, alleged the damage was caused by the administration of the incorrect mixture of drugs prior to the operation. The lawyer for the University of California, John S. Gilmore, maintained that Kevin White was a victim of a previously undiagnosed abnormality of the brain.

To win, Friedman was going to have to prove more than that Kevin White had been hurt while awaiting his intended operation. A bad outcome of treatment is not a sufficient proof of malpractice. Friedman also had to prove that the care provided to Kevin White was below the standard of care for heart surgery in the community. To prove this Friedman wanted Dean Mason to testify about what had happened.

And one morning in September 1984 he was trying to convince the judge to overrule the university's objections, and allow Mason to testify in front of the jury. Mason would tell the jury, Friedman said, that by 1977 "the cardiologists started to send patients away from the facility because . . . of the lack of competency of the surgeons."

The judge ruled that Mason could testify. He expected to take the stand after lunch to tell his story in public for the first time. He knew he could expect harsh cross-examination from the opposing lawyers.

But as the trial resumed, the lawyers for the university approached the bench. There was no need to continue. The parties had agreed to a settlement. It was later revealed that the university agreed to pay White $3.1 million immediately, and provide financial support for Kevin White's entire life, an amount which could conceivably total $40 million. The university would never risk another trial.

Joshua Davis was a four-year-old Sacramento boy who underwent the same operation for which Kevin White was scheduled. The surgeon was Edward J. Hurley. Davis suffered brain damage that rendered him subject to seizures and fits of abnormal behavior. Attorneys for Davis alleged that the brain damage resulted from an incorrect dosage of drugs soon after the operation. The case never went to trial, but the University of California agreed to pay $900,000 in damages and regular support payments for the remainder of Davis' life, payments which could total $36.9 million.

Linda Bish was a twelve-year-old girl with a congenital birth defect called the tetralogy of Fallot. Surgical repair of the defect involves two main steps. First, the surgeon uses a dacron patch to close the opening that had been permitting blood to pass from the right ventricle directly into the left ventricle, instead of being pumped to the lungs. Second, the surgeon must relieve any narrowing or obstruction in the pulmonary valve or nearby passages. When the right ventricle begins pumping at full capacity, the outflow passages must be open to accept the increased flow, or the heart may suffer irreparable damage. Linda Bish died of right heart failure following open-heart surgery at the university medical center. Her attorneys alleged that the surgeon, Edward J. Hurley, had not insured that the passages were fully clear. The University of California paid damages in the case, reportedly a large amount, but the total payment remained secret under terms of the settlement.

Alfred Clement, fifty-five, received three grafts in an elective coronary bypass operation supervised by Todd Grehl. Following the surgery an infection developed in the sternum which had been sawed open to perform the surgery. After the infection invaded the bone marrow Clement required additional surgery for removal of his sternum. The medical school paid damages in the case, but the amount was not revealed.

In all, the university paid damages in at least thirty-five other malpractice cases. How many millions of dollars in damage payments the episode in heart surgery ultimately cost has never been revealed.

16
NO COMPARISONS NEEDED

When the computer exercise first began there was no reason to suppose it would raise questions about heart surgery in Philadelphia. It was not even immediately evident why a U.S. Public Health Service physician named Henry Krakauer believed he had discovered an electronic version of Archimedes' famous lever. That was a bold vision for the tenant of a one-man office buried deep in the bowels of the government bureaucracy in Baltimore, and armed only with an inexpensive portable computer he had purchased himself. Krakauer is a slight man, almost painfully lean, with closely cropped brown hair and intense dark eyes. And while he would not have used allusions as grandiose as Archimedes, he was plainly excited, and grasped the potential impact of what he was doing. To understand it requires a brief expedition into the electronic backyard of the modern medical world.

Any patient who appears at a hospital in the United States is usually asked two specific questions before any detailed inquiry into what is wrong. The first is, "Do you have medical insurance?" The second request is for a nine-digit Social Security number. That number is the universal patient identification code for computerized medical records that are standardized on a national basis, especially for the 42 percent of all hospital bills that will be paid by the federal government. This is the Medicare population. Whether the patient leaves the hospital quickly, or after a prolonged stay, dead or alive, he will leave behind a standardized electronic record that will be collected on reels of magnetic tape. In each state these tapes ultimately pass into the hands of groups of medical analysts with the somewhat misleading name of Peer Review Organizations. These are private contractors in the employ of a giant but little known government agency called the Health Care Financing Administration, commonly abbreviated as HCFA and pronounced "Hick-Vah." With an eighty billion-dollar-a-year budget there is only one larger consumer of goods and services in the whole government, the Department of Defense. The first job of the Peer Review Organization is to try to save some of the taxpayers' money by limiting unnecessary hospitalization and rejecting improper hospital bills, using the data tapes and other information. The second task, almost a hopeless mission given their limited staff and money, is to make sure that care given to Medicare patients is of high quality.

The computer tapes, after being analyzed on the PRO computers, are forwarded to HCFA headquarters in Baltimore where they are entered into one of the most massive data bases in the country. So enormous is the master Medicare patient record file that if printed out in a continuous strip like the Dow Jones ticker, one year's records could be wrapped around the earth at the equator 263 times. And it was this enormous assemblage of medical experience that Krakauer could tap with his handy portable computer.

Krakauer had the position, the experience, and the training to grasp the opportunity. In addition to his M.D. he had a Ph.D. in chemistry, and was a self-taught computer programmer. He also held the rank equivalent to colonel in the U.S. Public Health Service. He had been detailed to the small HCFA agency in Baltimore that was responsible for supervising the state-level Peer Review Organizations. His job was to help the contracting firms devise programs to improve the quality of care for Medicare patients. The year was 1986, and Krakauer had an idea that would affect the actions, perspective, and thinking of every one of the 5,500 acute care hospitals in the United States. But it would turn out quite different than Krakauer had planned.

In the normal, day-to-day business of medicine there is a customary method for identifying and correcting mistakes in the diagnosis and treatment of patients, and it is taught early in every physician's training. A group of physicians in the same specialty and same hospital examine a patient chart, asking "Is there something we should have done differently in this case?" The reviewers have an enormous amount of detailed information about the patient, and they know intimately the hospital and physicians involved in the case. To encourage candor such sessions are legally secret, and any conclusions reached are rarely revealed outside the confines of the small group that sat around the table. The experiment that Henry Krakauer was going to undertake represented an approach that was diametrically opposite to case review, the conventional and accepted way of doing business.

Krakauer was going to examine every death among Medicare patients in every hospital in the country over one year's time. With his portable computer he would dial up HCFA's giant mainframe computers, and instruct them to create a separate file on every hospital in the country. Then he was going to compare their performance. Were Medicare patients much more likely to die in some hospitals than in others? Did some hospitals demonstrate extraordinary success among patients with life-threatening illnesses? He was going to examine overall mortality, after adjusting for many but not all of the differences in patients admitted to the various hospitals. He would also include nine separate diagnoses or surgical procedures. One of them was coronary bypass surgery.

This approach was strong at the exact point where case-by-case peer review is weakest. Seldom do physicians and hospitals ever compare their results with other institutions, and the individual case judgments are prone to be highly subjective. Krakauer was imposing the objective rigor of statistical theory, and comparisons between hospitals were the heart of his scheme. But the major weakness of Krakauer's approach happened to coincide with the one strong point of peer review: the wealth of clinical detail about each patient. It was a meager, stripped-down version of a patient chart that ultimately reached HCFA's computers. But Krakauer never planned to reach a medical judgment on individual cases, and was uncertain about just what conclusions might be reached about entire hospitals. The plan was to find out just what was going on. The results, a 102-page computer printout packed with columns of statistics about hundreds of hospitals, were to be sent to the state Peer Review Organizations to investigate. It is remarkable that just one public servant, operating without the assistance of so much as a secretary, devised this scheme, did all the necessary computer programming, selected the analytical techniques, and produced the finished analysis. It is equally surprising that such studies were not already being done on a routine basis. But there it was, one physician sitting astride an official river of computer data, and diverting some of the flow to a whole new useful purpose. It might even have turned out as the low-key professional exercise Krakauer planned had it not come to the attention of the news media.

• • •

MEDICINE WAS NOT specifically Joel Brinkley's beat in *The New York Times* Washington Bureau, but it was an interest. Brinkley had won a job at the *Times* in part because of his reporting for the *Louisville Courier-Journal* revealing dramatic weaknesses in the state of Kentucky's licensing of physicians. And it happened that one day Brinkley was at HCFA headquarters inquiring what this federal agency was doing to fulfill its legal responsibility to insure that Medicare patients were protected from poor medical care. That is the primary responsibility of a small HCFA agency called the Bureau of Health Standards and Quality, and Brinkley ended up in the office of its director, Philip Nathanson.

During the course of an interview about the bureau's activities, Nathanson happened to describe Krakauer's study of hospitals with high and low death rates, which was known officially as a "Model for the Prediction of Statistical Outliers."

"This has never been done before," Nathanson told Brinkley. "Like any kind of statistical data, this doesn't necessarily mean there is a problem."

When Nathanson would not release Krakauer's study, in particular the names of the hospitals, Brinkley turned on the heat. He soon had written a story headlined U.S. DISTRIBUTING LISTS OF HOSPITALS WITH UNUSUAL DEATH RATES.

"The Department of Health and Human Services is sending state agencies lists of hospitals whose death rates, or rates of complications, exceed the national average," Brinkley wrote.

His story about Krakauer's study had the intended effect of announcing the existence of the list to the world at large, and HCFA was soon deluged with hundreds of demands for the specific hospital names. In a matter of days the agency reversed its position, and released with little preparation and explanation Krakauer's complex analysis, a study that had never been intended for public consumption.

It was clumsy. It was unplanned. Even the cover page of the HCFA release backed away from the study with a full page of reasons why high mortality rates might not suggest inadequate care. And it was not exactly greeted by cries of approval from the key players in the medical world.

"It's the dumbest thing I've ever seen H.H.S. do," said Jack Owen, executive vice-president of the American Hospital Association.

Nevertheless it was the beginning of a new era. No longer would the questions of the quality of care be reserved to the secrecy of the peer review process. The government was making comparisons between hospitals, naming names for the first time ever. And it was going to affect hospitals from coast to coast.

• • •

ONE OF THOSE lists soon reached the hands of Gilbert M. Gaul, a reporter for the *Philadelphia Inquirer.* He found one comparison between two medical schools so striking that it became the lead of his story.

Located right in Philadelphia was the Medical College of Pennsylvania, and according to Krakauer's study, it had performed fifty coronary bypass operations on Medicare patients in 1984. Twenty percent of these patients had died, a total of ten deaths. On the same page of the same list were the results for another medical school, Emory University in Atlanta. At Emory just eight patients died in 448 bypass operations, for a mortality rate of 1.8 percent. Given the same specific surgical procedure undertaken on patients of similar age, how could one hospital have a death rate ten times higher than the other? Had Emory posted such impressive results over just ten or twenty operations, it would be easy to suspect a statistical fluke, or perhaps an unusual group of patients. But it does not take elaborate statistical theory to sense that the law of averages is going to catch up with Emory University over the course of nearly 500 bypass operations. The same compelling logic seemed to apply to the Medical College of Pennsylvania. Even if it experienced no deaths in its next fifty bypass operations, the hospital would still be left with a 10 percent mortality rate. Even a 10 percent death rate would not be confidence-inspiring when compared to Emory's 1.8 percent. So Gaul interviewed the Medical College of Pennsylvania's hospital administrator, JoAnn Mower, to inquire into the reasons for the results.

"We get many patients between the ages of sixty-five and eighty-five who have multiple illnesses, and are more complex to treat," explained Mower. The figures did not take risk or severity into account, she said.

Mower's explanation, however, was only the opening salvo in a more extensive assault on the HCFA data. Next came a detailed letter-to-the-editor from Bernard Sigel, the college's chief of surgery, attacking both the accuracy of the figures, and appropriateness of Gaul's comparison.

"My hospital, Medical College of Pennsylvania, as part of a medical school complex, treats the most serious and emergent clinical problems," wrote Sigel. "And yet the government, and consequently your article, attempts to compare a facility like ours with others, which although performing large numbers of the procedure, may be operating only on less severe cases."

Sigel also claimed that not only was the comparison wrong, the data was wrong. The hospital had operated on eighty-four Medicare patients, not fifty, and only seven died. That was an 8.3 percent mortality rate, not the 20 percent reported by the government, Sigel said.

The hospital did not let the matter rest with a letter to the editor. It continued to assail the HCFA study in a full-page advertisement entitled, THE HEART OF THE MATTER IS THE QUALITY OF CARE.

"The government's figures are flawed and inaccurate," it said. "They reveal only a small part of the total picture, and even that is distorted. The figures pose a national problem for hospitals and, in our case, they plainly misrepresent the quality of care."

The hospital's immediate concern, hospital officials said later, was the impact of the disclosures on their competitive position. Open-heart surgery was performed at ten other hospitals in Philadelphia, and it might not take much to shift large numbers of patients to other institutions. After the hospital had dealt with the competitive threat; after it had assured the public about the high quality of its cardiac care; and after it had denounced the HCFA data as inaccurate, then and only then did it begin an inquiry into the deaths in its cardiac surgery program. Until Krakauer's analysis they had noticed nothing amiss.

It soon emerged that the HCFA figures were a more accurate reflection of the medical college's mortality experience than the chief of surgery's own numbers. The 8.3 percent mortality rate Sigel had cited in his letter to the editor was incorrect. The HCFA figures had omitted some of the bypass operations. When all the cases were included, the mortality rate was 18.5 percent among Medicare patients, quite close to the 20 percent in Krakauer's study. Furthermore the results were not a chance occurrence, or the result of some temporary aberration. When the hospital tallied a second year's operative experience, the results were virtually identical: an 18.9 percent mortality rate. As the hospital had argued so loudly, however, a mortality rate by itself may not be meaningful without a separate examination of how severely ill the patients were at the time of bypass surgery. And when Sigel and other members of the faculty began to examine the cases from this perspective they soon concluded that their results were not only acceptable but readily explained.

Sigel divided all the Medicare patients into two groups. If they were uncomplicated bypass operations performed on an elective basis, the patient was placed in the low/moderate risk group. But if, for example, the operation was classified as emergency surgery, the patient was placed in the high-risk group. If the left ventricle was damaged to the point that it could only pump out half or less of the blood that filled the chamber, the patient was also classified as high risk. If low cardiac output had created other symptoms—for example, fluid in the lungs— the patient was also placed in the high-risk group. Finally any patient over seventy-five years old was automatically classified as high risk. And when the hospital's Medicare patients were thus grouped more than half of them fell into the high-risk category. And when Sigel examined the charts of the Medicare patients who had died, he found that practically all of them had one or more risk factors, and some had several. Thus Sigel and his surgical colleagues at the Medical College of Pennsylvania were satisfied, as were the chairman of the department of medicine, the vice-president for clinical affairs, and the chancellor.

What is striking about the medical college's analysis is the extent to which it entirely ignored the whole point of the HCFA study. Sigel's risk groups were logical, but they did not constitute an accepted scheme used in any other medical institution, let alone a previously published scientific study. More importantly, to learn that most of their deaths had occurred among patients classified as "high risk" should not have reassured the medical college physicians, any more than an airline management should be relieved to learn that most of its recent crashes occurred during bad weather or during other difficulties. The whole thrust of the HCFA study was to suggest that the medical college's mortality rate was unusually high in comparison with other hospitals. And the risk factor analysis does not survive even the crudest comparisons with other institutions. Some examples:

A simple ranking by Medicare mortality rate shows that of the 494 United States hospitals performing at least thirty bypass operations, 491 of them had lower mortality rates than the medical college. The comparison does not become much more favorable if the medical college is allowed to exclude the one half of its patients it classified as high risk. Among the remainder 11 percent died following bypass surgery. The national average among Medicare patients in 1984 was 5.5 percent, and included all the high-risk patients in other hospitals.

The medical college's record does not look any stronger when patients of all ages are considered, rather than just the over-sixty-five Medicare population. Overall, the hospital said it experienced an 11 percent mortality rate among patients of all ages. That was almost four times higher than the average for all New York State hospitals in 1984, which was 3.2 percent. It was more than five times higher than the 1.9 percent mortality rate for all bypass operations in metropolitan Washington, D.C. And no Washington area hospital had a mortality rate above 3.2 percent. Even if one were to suppose that the Medical College of Pennsylvania operated on twice as many high-risk patients as any hospital in Washington, or all of them combined, the comparison would still be unfavorable. The real tragedy is not that the Medical

College of Pennsylvania could not immediately explain these enormous discrepancies, but that it did not even notice them.

The Medical College of Pennsylvania was of course not the only medical institution to be affected by Henry Krakauer's first tentative pull on the lever of change. The chief cardiac surgeon at a San Francisco hospital found himself explaining his high mortality rate on a national television show (sicker patients, he said). On WNBC-TV news similar comparisons were made between the mortality rates in bypass surgery at two New York City hospitals. By the next year consulting firms were sponsoring conferences and providing computer analyses of hospital mortality data using HCFA data. Robert Steinbrook of the *Los Angeles Times* published lengthy studies of the mortality rates in California for bypass surgery for both 1985 and 1986. One hospital, Eisenhower Medical Center in Rancho Mirage, even took out a full-page advertisement in the *Wall Street Journal* to announce that its mortality rate for bypass surgery was lowest among all hospitals performing 150 or more operations a year on Medicare patients. The ad was greeted by considerable outrage in medical circles, a reaction that is somewhat hard to understand given that most medical advertising about quality of care generally doesn't have any factual basis whatsoever. Despite a chorus of complaints from the industry, the Health Care Financing Administration continued to improve both the quality and quantity of comparative information it released about hospitals. But it was still too early to tell whether this data was the beginning of a transformation of the way medicine does business, or just a ripple on the waters of business as usual.

UNCERTAIN OUTCOMES

The successes in medical care for the human heart described in this book are primarily triumphs of teamwork and technology. They portray a vital community of committed researchers and practitioners who are far from fallible, but commendably open to new ideas. A surprisingly simple idea links most of the criticisms: Far too little attention, time, and money are invested in measuring the outcomes of medical care.

Millions undergo hazardous treatment of undetermined benefit because the proper controlled studies were never performed. It is unlikely that the public would tolerate the marginal performance of emergency medical services in many communities if a count were kept of how many lives were needlessly forfeited each month from cardiac arrest. We cannot accurately measure either gains or losses in the health status of the nation because physicians are sloppy, and the government lax about death certificates and other vital statistics. Because hospitals do not routinely compare their results in open-heart surgery with other institutions, they remain unaware of serious failings. All these problems spring from a lack of systematic information about what happens to patients as a result of treatment, because of inattention to the outcomes of medical care.

Too often the fragmentary information that does exist is not assessed objectively. The misguided decisions on cholesterol doubtless occurred because a small circle of influential physicians got too close to their subject, and bet their careers on a single narrow approach to preventing coronary heart disease. Cardiologists and surgeons became so deeply committed to bypass surgery that they could not appreciate the mounting evidence that the benefits of the procedure were significantly limited. The secret insider government of peer review invites arbitrary and subjective judgments that, as we have seen, are often tragically flawed.

This lack of information has the unintended effect of depriving all patients of the fundamental right of informed consent. The most conscientious physician cannot provide a patient with a fair statement of the risks and benefits of treatment if these have never been determined. One has to admire Michael DeBakey's courage in performing the early carotid endarterectomy, but marvel at his hubris in informing the patient that the risks of an operation that he had never performed before were "slight." It is a favorite aphorism of heart surgeons that surgery is appropriate even when the prospects of survival are slim, provided that the risks of the operation are smaller than the risks of taking no action. That might be a reasonable proposition provided that risks of either course of action were actually known.

But can medicine afford a more open system? This book was written with full awareness that the cold and calculating candor with which medical treatments were assessed would prove deeply disturbing to some patients, and provoke angry denunciations from some physicians. Patients with a terrifying heart condition may desperately want simple and reassuring answers. The facts in this book are neither simple or reassuring, and may directly undermine the faith and optimism that form one of the mysterious and unmeasurable ways that doctors help patients get better. At the extreme, books such as Bernie S. Siegel's immensely popular *Love, Medicine and Miracles* seem to suggest that a positive mental attitude towards health and medicine somehow transcends the mundane effects of a specific treatment. Forget about statistics and believe you're going to be the exception, Siegel counsels his readers.

That might be viable advice to his main audience, patients with life-threatening diseases. But it is a disastrous prescription for how to improve a system for medical care that increasingly resorts to technically demanding and potentially hazardous treatments.

One person who put these complex forces in clear perspective was the thoughtful scientist, physician and author, Lewis Thomas. In *The Youngest Science* he describes his earliest perceptions of medicine, formed while accompanying his father on house calls in the early decades of this century. Physicians spent a lot of time talking to patients, he recalled, because often that was the only treatment that was available.

"Patients do get better," Thomas wrote, "some of them anyway, from even the worst diseases; there are very few illnesses, like rabies, that kill all comers. Most of them tend to kill some patients and spare others, and if you are one of the lucky ones and have also at hand a steady and knowledgeable doctor, you become convinced that the doctor saved you.

"My father's early instructions to me, sitting in the front of his car on his rounds, was that I should be careful not to believe this of myself if I become a doctor."

FACTUAL SOURCES

Articles in the medical literature are referred to by publication, year, volume, and beginning page number. Example: *Circulation* (1988) 312:102. In the text journal articles are usually attributed to the first-listed author even though many list multiple authors. Books are cited by author and title only; complete information can be found in the Bibliography. Drugs are usually referred to by their generic name rather than the manufacturer's registered brand name. An Appendix includes both names. In virtually every instance quotations in the book are verbatim excerpts of tape-recorded interviews, or from official transcripts, court documents, or sworn depositions. Quotations from official records, tape recordings of public meetings, or court documents were regarded as sufficiently authoritative as not to require a further interview; in some instances individuals quoted in the book from official records declined to be interviewed. The names of physicians, hospitals, and patients are real unless specifically noted. The names of two medical journals are abbreviated, the *New England Journal of Medicine (New Eng Jnl Med)* and *Journal of the American Medical Association (JAMA)*. The National Heart, Lung, and Blood Institute is abbreviated as NHLBI.

1. Two Patients, Two Outcomes

The accuracy of the exercise stress test, and the lower reliability for women, was from *Cardiology for the House Officer.* The cost was typical of Washington Metropolitan area hospitals in 1988. Angioplasty failure rates are discussed in detail in Chapter 8. The effect of failed angioplasty on cardiac surgery mortality rates was examined in *Journal of Thoracic and Cardiovascular Surgery* (1986) 92:847, and the *Annals of Thoracic Surgery* (1985) 40:7.

The proportions of deaths by cause were from the National Center for Health Statistics, *Monthly Vital Statistics Report,* July 29, 1988, for the classifications "diseases of the heart" and "malignant neoplasms." The figures were for calendar 1987. The cost of bypass surgery was based on an annual volume of 230,000 operations per year. Bypass surgery cost estimates vary considerably depending on whether costs of cardiac catheterization and follow-up care were included. Costs for space exploration were from Account 253, Space Flight, in the *Budget of the United States Government,* Fiscal Year 1988.

The massive decline in the death rate for coronary heart disease was examined in the *Proceedings of the Conference on the Decline in Coronary Heart Disease Mortality,* NIH Publication No. 79-160, 1979. Thomas Thom's comments were made at the December 7, 1986 NHLBI workshop in the paper, "Trends and Determinants of Coronary Heart Disease Mortality." Jeff Maurer was a coauthor.

The Veterans Administration Cooperative Study Group reported the dramatic results of the severe hypertension trial (115 to 129 mm Hg diastolic) in *JAMA* (1967) 202:116. A report on the second cohort, with less severe hypertension (90 to 114 mm Hg) appeared in *JAMA* (1970) 213:1143. Examples of the debate on mild hypertension were in *JAMA* (1983) 250:3171 and *New Eng Jnl Med* (1982) 307:307. The estimate of persons on blood pressure medication was from NHLBI, "Hypertension Prevalence and the Status of Awareness, Treatment, and Control in the United States, 1985." Hypertension medication estimates were based on the monthly retail cost in Washington of mid-priced medication for mild hypertension. The complication rate was from a recent British trial of mild hypertension, reported in *British Med Jnl* (1985) 291:97. Adverse effects were further explored in *New Eng Jnl Med* (1986) 314:1657. The psychological research on patient adherence was summarized in "Patient Compliance to Prescribed Antihypertensive Medication Regimens," *NIH Publication No. 81-2102*, October 1980.

Michael DeBakey described his first carotid endarterectomy in *JAMA* (1975) 233:1083. The historical record on who performed the "first" such operation is not exactly clear. The earliest known operation on the carotid was performed in 1949 by Francis Murphey, for many years a professor of neurosurgery at Harvard. The Cincinnati area mortality and complication rates appeared in *Stroke* (1984) 15:950. The Rand Corporation study was published in *New Eng Jnl Med* (1988) 318:721. The American Neurological Association's committee conclusions appeared in the *Annals of Neurology* (1987) 22:72. An inconclusive clinical trial appeared in *JAMA* (1970) 211:1993, where again potential benefits were offset by high mortality and morbidity. A more recent British trial also failed to demonstrate benefits, and appeared in *Journal of the Neurological Sciences* (1984) 64:45.

The figures for Medicare patient mortality in bypass surgery were calculated by the author from a computer tape released by the Health Care Financing Administration and confirmed by the two hospitals. Eugene Wallsh was interviewed by Michael York, then a colleague at Knight-Ridder, Inc. Jack R. Steinlieb was interviewed by the author. The new surgical team at Lenox Hill was announced in an Oct. 12, 1987, press release. The 1988 results among 107 Medicare patients for isolated CABG were courtesy of Lenox Hill Hospital.

2. Hearts Then and Now

The basic embryology and anatomy of the human heart were ably portrayed in the traditional reference, *Anatomy of the Human Body* by Henry Gray. The historical material was assembled from various medical histories, among them Erwin H. Ackerknecht's *A Short History of Medicine,* P.E. Baldry's *The Battle Against Heart Disease; Discovers of Blood Circulation* by T. Doby, and *The History of Coronary Heart Disease* by J.O. Leibowitz. Vesalius' quote came from Doby, and Hippocrates' description of a heart attack came from Leibowitz. The operations of the electrical system and other aspects of physiology of the heart were explained in Arthur C. Guyton's *Textbook of Medical Physiology.* Animal comparisons came from *Comparative Anatomy of the Vertebrates* by George C. Kent, and *Comparative Vertebrate Anatomy* by Marvalee H. Wake. The fundamentals were illuminated and explained by Professors Richard S. Snell and David L. Atkins of George Washington University.

3. The Campaign Begins

A one-page handout, "National Cholesterol Education Program: Goals and Objectives," describes the overall plan. Full details appear in the benchmark document for the program, "Report of the Expert Panel on Detection, Evaluation and Treatment of High Blood Cholesterol in Adults," October 5, 1987. The numbers of people affected were estimates of James I. Cleeman, program coordinator. Costs of previous research came from the *NHLBI Fact Book,* Fiscal Year 1986.

The original Korean War report appeared in *JAMA* (1953) 152:1090. A reprint and historical retrospective appeared thirty years later in *JAMA* (1983) 256:2863. Details of the clinical manifestations of coronary heart disease were culled from various cardiology texts, especially J. Willis Hurst's *The Heart.*

Thomas R. Dawber describes the epidemiological project in his 1980 book, *The Framingham Study.* The NHLBI also publishes a bibliography of Framingham research that at last count had generated 433 scholarly articles. The historical example on cholera was from John P. Fox's *Epidemiology, Man and Disease.* The table showing the incidence of coronary heart disease in the Framingham study was calculated by the author from the public-use computer tape of the study

at the twenty-year mark. These results, which average all ten cholesterol readings, were considerably more modest than more widely
quoted figures which either are limited to men, or based on a single
cholesterol measurement (usually the second) or both. Using only the
early second measurement introduces bias because the cholesterol/
heart disease relationship deteriorates later in life. The Framingham
diet study appears as Section 24 among a multi-volume series of papers
and tables that never got published in the referred medical journals.
The series is: "The Framingham Study: an Epidemiological Investigation of Cardiovascular Disease," *DHEW Pub. No. (NIH) 74-618,
74-478, 74-599, 76-1083.*

The task force published its findings in "Arteriosclerosis: A Report
by the National Heart Lung, and Blood Institute Task Force on Arteriosclerosis," June 1971, *DHEW Pub. No. (NIH) 72-137.* A working
group has published updated findings at intervals until the present day.

4. CHOLESTEROL ON TRIAL

The MR.FIT original design, and the methods used to reduce risk
factors were described in six consecutive articles in *Preventive Medicine*
(1981) 10:387. The effects of diet were further outlined in the *Journal
of the American Dietetic Association* (1986) 86:744 & 752. The final
results appeared in *JAMA* (1982) 248:1465.

The investigators' original design for the cholesterol drug trial was
published in the *Journal of Chronic Disease* (1979) 32:609. The final
results appeared in *JAMA* (1984) 251:351. An example of how the
results were sold to the medical community appeared in the *American
Journal of Cardiology* (1984) 54:30C. The clofibrate trial results were
reported in the *British Heart Journal* (1978) 40:1069. The sad story of
the Coronary Drug Project appeared in the following articles: *JAMA*
(1970) 214:1301; *JAMA* (1972) 220:996; *JAMA* (1973) 226:652;
JAMA (1975) 231:360. Geoffrey Rose describes the clofibrate problem
in the *International Journal of Epidemiology* (1985) 14:32. Two critical
assessments of the CPPT appeared in the same issue of *JAMA* (1985)
254:2091 and 2094.

The theory behind the inappropriate use of the one-tailed test appeared in Robert W. Woolson's *Statistical Methods for the Analysis of Biomedical Data,* page 132-133. A parallel example was in Bourke, *Interpretation and Uses of Medical Statistics,* page 77, where the authors concluded: "For instance, it would be dangerous if the researchers assumed, prior to the study, that the drug would only have a beneficial effect on survival."

Nine years after the Coronary Drug Project ended the heart institute conducted a follow-up study that showed a reduction in total mortality among those who had taken niacin. But it is impossible to determine whether the benefit came from taking niacin or discontinuing it. A report appears in the *Journal of the American College of Cardiology* (1986) 8:1245.

5. A DANGEROUS CONDITION

The account of the Consensus Development Conference was based on a tape recording of the session provided courtesy of the National Institutes of Health, Division of External Affairs, and on abstracts and the conference consensus statement. Another observer's report on the conference was Gina Kolata's account in *Science* (1984) 227:40, which was also the source of the quote of Thomas Chalmers. The events were further explored in interviews with Basil M. Rifkind, Edward H. Ahrens, Jr., and Eliot Corday. The final consensus statement was published in *JAMA* (1985) 253:2080.

The first description of the campaign appears in the American Heart Association's "Rationale of Heart–Diet Statement," published in *Circulation* (1982) 64:839A. The 1983 physician's poll was published in *JAMA* (1987) 258:3521. Claude Lenfant's statements to the NHLBI's advisory council were from transcripts of the sessions.

The prime source for the many details of the cholesterol education program was the lengthy report of the expert panel cited in Chapter 3. The comments from James I. Cleeman were from an interview. The American Medical Association's campaign was announced in *JAMA* (1988) 260:3195. (Note that page numbers don't actually appear in the advertisement.) The role of the other participants was reported by Michael Waldholz in the *Wall Street Journal,* Dec. 6, 1988, page B6.

The interlocking directorate of the cholesterol establishment was gleaned from the conference and publication statements cited above. The lovastatin physician's network was described by Merck in an enclosure to the Sept. 1, 1987, press release announcing the FDA approval of the drug.

The details of laboratory measurement problems were revealed in "Current Status of Blood Cholesterol Measurement in Clinical Laboratories in the United States," a report from the Laboratory Standardization Panel of the National Cholesterol Education Program, draft report of Sept. 29, 1987. A later survey of laboratories in the northwest was published in *Clinical Chemistry* (1988) 8:1629. Walt Bogdanich's Pulitzer Prize-winning articles on the shortcomings of clinical laboratories described his cholesterol tests, and was published in the *Wall Street Journal,* Feb. 2–3, 1987. The experience of the Tennessee employees was reported in the *American Journal of Medical Science* (1988) 295(1):11. D.M. Hegsted and Robert J. Nicolosi reported on individual cholesterol variation in *Proceedings of the National Academy of Sciences* (1987) 84:6259. Problems of HDL measurement were reported in *JAMA* (1986) 256:2714, and in the northwest clinical laboratory survey cited above. Calculations of misclassification were based on two standard deviations from the mean, the standard suggested by Hegsted. Basil M. Rifkind's comments were from a tape-recorded interview. At this writing the effect of a new law passed in 1988 regulating clinical laboratories is uncertain.

The heart–diet trial was rejected by the National Heart, Lung, and Blood Institute Task Force on Arteriosclerosis report cited in Chapter 3. The Framingham, Puerto Rico and Honolulu diet and heart disease experience was reported in *Circulation* (1981) 63:500. William P. Castelli's examination of alcohol appeared in *Lancet* (1977) 2:153. Ancel Keys' international study, "Coronary Heart Disease in Seven Countries," was a book-length supplement to the journal *Circulation* published in 1970.

The INTERSALT study of salt consumption in thirty-two countries was reported in the *British Medical Journal* (1988) 297(6644):319.

William Ira Bennett's comment was in his "Body and Mind" column in *The New York Times Magazine,* Jan. 22, 1989, page 30. An example of the longstanding skepticism of the international comparison was M. Gary Nicholls' review of the literature on salt in *Hypertension* (1984) 6:795.

The Heart–Diet Pilot was published in a *Circulation* supplement (1968) 37:I-1. The MR.FIT results were cited in Chapter 4. The Northwestern study appeared in the *Journal of the American Dietetic Association* (1986) 86:759. Despite all the tremendous interest in the cholesterol-lowering properties of oat bran this was the only reference involving free-living humans in the entire scientific literature, according to a computer search of abstracts. The statistically non-significant results have been repeatedly reported as scientific evidence for oat bran's efficacy. The authors claim the pooled results to pass a one-tailed test of significance, but the straightforward test, as shown in Table 2, page 762, shows an enormous variation in individual response and non-significant results. Oat bran might work, but the proper studies have yet to demonstrate it. The diet component of the cholesterol drug trial was described in the main studies cited in Chapter 4, although it should be observed that diet responders were specifically excluded. The Robert I. Levy and Daniel Steinberg quotations were from the consensus conference tapes, James I. Cleeman's from a tape-recorded interview.

6. THE DANGERS OF LOW CHOLESTEROL

Geoffrey Rose and colleagues reported their unexpected findings on cholesterol and colon cancer in *Lancet* (1974) 1:181. The French report appeared in the *American Journal of Epidemiology* (1980) 112:-388. The Framingham data confirming the relationship was published in the *Journal of the National Cancer Institute* (1982) 69:989, and the Health Examination and Nutrition Survey appeared first in *Lancet* (1987) 2:298. The Veterans trial report on polyunsaturated fat and diet appeared in *Lancet* (1971) 1:464, and the incidence of gallstones in that trial was reported in *New Eng Jnl Med* (1976) 288:24. The Japanese reported the relationship between low cholesterol and stroke in *Preventive Medicine* (1979) 8:104, and extensive rebuttal and cautionary notes appeared immediately thereafter.

The NHLBI discussions of whether to conduct a trial of lovastatin, and the comment on compactin appeared in the transcript of its Advisory Council meeting, September 10, 1987. The NHLBI position on the long-term safety of lovastatin appears in the adult treatment guidelines of the National Cholesterol Education Program, op. cit. Chapter 3. The little-known saga of triparanol is told in Ralph Fine's book, *The Great Drug Deception.* Rifkind's comments about compactin were made at an Advisory Council meeting. The human and animal side effects, and Saul Genuth's comments appear in the transcript of the FDA advisory committee on endocrinologic and metabolic drugs on February 19, 1987. The initial multi-center trial of lovastatin was reported in *JAMA* (1986) 256:2928; the cholestyramine comparison in *JAMA* (1988) 260:359. Scott Grundy's assessment of synthesis inhibitors (of which lovastatin was the only available drug) appeared in *New Eng Jnl Med* (1988) 319:24. Responses, including the report on sleep effects, appeared in *New Eng Jnl Med* (1988) 319:1222. Other side effects were reported in *New Eng Jnl Med* (1988) 318:46.

The Helsinki trial of gemfibrozil was reported in *New Eng Jnl Med* (1987) 317:1237; Basil M. Rifkind's analysis appeared in the same issue at page 1279.

Jeremiah Stamler's initial spin-off of the MR.FIT study (without total mortality) appeared in *JAMA* (1986) 256:2823. Total mortality by cholesterol decile was disclosed in one of the tables of an article examining cholesterol and cancer in *JAMA* (1987) 257:948. James C. Taylor's analysis of cholesterol reduction and life expectancy appeared in the *Annals of Internal Medicine* (1987) 106:605. A rebuttal from William Castelli et al. appears in the *Annals of Internal Medicine* (1988) 108:313. The Framingham study examination of life expectancy appeared in *JAMA* (1987) 257:2176. The changes in the nation's serum cholesterol levels were plotted through the National

Health and Nutrition Examination Surveys and reported in *JAMA* (1978) 257:937. Here are some further overviews of the cholesterol question from the medical literature: Michael Oliver offered two of the most detailed critiques, one on strategies in *Circulation* (1986) 73:1, and another on the clinical trials in *Journal of the American College of Cardiology* (1988) 12:814. Salim Yusif provided a somewhat more optimistic meta-analysis in *JAMA* (1988) 260:2259. The National Cholesterol Education Program specifically was examined in the *Mayo Clinic Proceedings* (1988) 63:88. Robert M. Kaplan looked at cholesterol and other risk factors in a lengthy analysis in *Medical Care* (1985) 23:564. William Harlan examined the problems raised by cholesterol lowering in *JAMA* (1985) 253:2087. Marshall Becker's comments about the *Titanic* appeared in his review of the cholesterol question in the *Annals of Internal Medicine* (1988) 106:623.

7. A Lot Can Go Wrong

The bypass operation was observed by the author in May 1986. Heart surgeons are increasingly using the internal mammary arteries in the operation, which Jorge Garcia did not in this instance.

The details of the diagnosis and treatment of angina pectoris were taken primarily from J. Willis Hurst's and Noble O. Fowler's cardiology texts. The early history of heart surgery was reported in several surveys, especially "Research Progress in Surgery of Coronary Occlusive Disease," in the *Journal of Surgical Research* (1967) 7:188, and "Surgical Procedures to Revascularize the Heart," *American Journal of Surgery*, (1960) 100:572. Leonard Cobb's famous study of ligation of the internal mammary arteries was in *New Eng Jnl Med* (1959) 260:115. J.R. Kitchell's results were in *American Journal of Cardiology* (1958) 12:46, and I.C. Brill's in *Northwest Medicine* (1958) 57:483. The prolific Arthur Vineberg reported his results in numerous articles, examples being the *American Heart Journal* (1957) 54:851, and the *Annals of Surgery* (1964) 159:185. The Johns Hopkins study of pigs and dogs appeared in the *Journal of Thoracic Surgery* (1958) 35:699. Somewhat better results were obtained at the

University of Virginia, and reported in the *Journal of Thoracic and Cardiovascular Surgery* (1970) 59:774. F. Mason Sones described his discovery of a method of coronary angiography in a letter to Spencer King at Emory University, reprinted in King's book, *Coronary Arteriography and Angioplasty*.

The first major report of the Veterans Administration Cooperative Trial appeared in *New Eng Jnl Med* (1977) 297:621, and Eugene Braunwald's editorial comment appeared at page 661. The initial reaction to the findings was printed in the journal two months later beginning at (1977) 297:1462. The subset of patients (with left main coronary artery) was reported in a supplement to *Circulation* (1976): 54:Suppl 3:III-107. The effort to omit the high mortality centers appeared in *Circulation* (1982) 65:Suppl 2:II-60. The eleven-year follow-up was reported in *New Eng Jnl Med* (1984) 311:1335.

The main findings of the European Coronary Surgery Study Group appeared in *Lancet* (1982) 2:1173. A preview was published in *Circulation* (1982) 65:Suppl2:II-67, and the twelve-year follow-up appeared in *New Eng Jnl Med* (1988) 319:332.

The Coronary Artery Surgery Study (CASS) spawned scores of publications. The randomized-trial portion was reported in *Circulation* (1983) 68:939, and in more detail in *New Eng Jnl Med* (1984) 310:750. Michael DeBakey's criticism appeared in *JAMA* (1984) 252:2609. J. Ward Kennedy's analysis of surgical mortality in bypass surgery appeared in greatest and most interesting detail in the *Journal of Thoracic and Cardiovascular Surgery* (1980) 80:886.

The death rates and complications came from these sources: The 1986 mortality rate in California came from Robert Steinbrook's analysis of all procedures published in the *Los Angeles Times*, July 24, 1988, page 3, estimates of myocardial infarctions were contained in Rand Corporation's literature summary, "Indications for Selected Medical Surgical Procedures—a Literature Review and Ratings of Appropriateness," May 1986, the readmission rate figures came from a report in *Journal of the American Medical Association* (1985) 253:3568, and from an unpublished Health Care Financing Administration analysis.

8. No Trial Balloon

The example of angioplasty was observed by the author in September 1988.

Andreas Gruentzig's educational background came from his C.V., provided through courtesy of Emory University. C.F. Dotter was credited with inventing angioplasty in numerous accounts, for example, Spencer King's *Coronary Arteriography and Angioplasty*, which also included Gruentzig's report on his first case. The comments of Kenneth M. Kent, Peter C. Block, and Robert Reis were from taped interviews. J. Willis Hurst's tribute to Gruentzig in *Circulation* (1986) 73:606 included numerous personal details as did various other materials provided by Emory. Complications of PTCA were reported in *Circulation* (1983) 67:723, *Circulation* (1984)53:Suppl3:12C, 17C and 22C. Investigator experience was examined in the same supplement, 56C, and in the *American Heart Journal* (1984) 104:1019. An updated comparison of the original registry and more recent cases appeared in *New Eng Jnl Med* (1988) 318:265. The new guidelines for angioplasty appeared in the *Journal of the American College of Cardiology* (1988) 12:529. The physician salary figures were provided by the American Medical Association's Center for Health Policy Research, (Socioeconomic Characteristics of Medical Practice), 1987. Emilio Giuliani's comment appeared in the *Journal of the American College of Cardiology* (1985) 6:992. Restenosis is discussed in two editorial summaries in *Annals of Thoracic Surgery* (1985) 40:1 and *Journal of the American College of Cardiology* (1986) 8:6. The follow-up on Gruentzig's original cases appeared in *New Eng Jnl Med* (1987):316:1127. The potential of fish oil for reducing restenosis was suggested in *New Eng Jnl Med* (1988) 319:734.

9. A Mirror for Medicine

The details of President Eisenhower's heart attack were taken from *The New York Times*, editions of September 27 through October 10, 1955, and from Paul Dudley White's book, *My Life in Medicine*. The idea for using Eisenhower's heart attack as a benchmark to trace the evolution of treatment first appeared in Gregory D. Curfman's excellent analysis in the *New Eng Jnl Med* (1988) 318:1123. The heart attack figures for 1987 were from "Detailed Diagnoses and Surgical Procedures for Patients discharged from Short Stay Hospitals," 1987. The decline in inpatient mortality is discussed in W. B. Kannel's and Thomas J. Thom's "Implications of the declining mortality rate of cardiovascular diseases in the USA," appearing in *Recent Advances in Cardiology*. The intensity and cost of modern therapy were examined by Eric Sawitz in *JAMA* (1988) 259:2419.

The extent of unrecognized heart attacks was first revealed in a landmark Framingham paper, appearing in the *Annals of Internal Medicine* (1959) 50:1359. The failure to diagnose fatal heart attacks was described in *JAMA* (1983) 250:1177.

Claude S. Beck described the first electrical defibrillation in *JAMA* (1947) 135:985. The invention of CPR at Johns Hopkins was reported in *JAMA* (1960) 174:226. Hughes W. Day describes his first coronary care unit in *Diseases of the Chest* (1963) 44:423. Kenneth Brown's early Toronto experience was reported in *Lancet* (1963) 2:349

A British view of the history and development of coronary care units can be found in D. G. Julian's account in the *British Heart Journal* (1987) 57:497. Examples of how frequently arrhythmias were discovered appeared in the *American Journal of Cardiology* (1967) 20:451. Thomas Killip's early experiences were reported in *American Journal of Cardiology* (1967) 20:457. The results of the federal government's conference on coronary care units appeared as "Proceedings of the National Conference on Coronary Care Units," *DHEW Pub. No. 1764*, 1968. The quote from the *British Medical Journal* was from Julian's history, op. cit.

H.G. Mather's first study of home care for heart attacks appeared in the *British Medical Journal* (1971) 3:334; the second in the same publication (1976) 1:925. A. G. Hill's similar trial was published in *Lancet* (1978) 1:837. A United States perspective appeared in *JAMA* (1984) 251:349. Geoffrey Rose's assessment of coronary care was in the *British Journal of Preventive Social Medicine* (1975) 29:147, and

Thomas Thom's assessment of the decline in case fatality rate in his chapter, op.cit. The prophylactic use of lidocaine was assessed in *JAMA* (1988) 260:1910 and *JAMA* (1988) 260:2088. The frequency of ventricular fibrillation among heart attack patients in coronary care units came from Lee Goldman's assessment of the decline in coronary heart disease mortality in the *Annals of Internal Medicine* (1984) 101:825, and was calculated from the *JAMA* study of prophylactic lidocaine, op.cit. Ostler Peterson's criticism of the studies of Hughes Day and others appeared in the *Annals of Internal Medicine* (1976) 85:819, and the Peterson and Bloom study on the utilization of intensive care units was in *New Eng Jnl Med* (1973) 288:72. David M. Siegel's excellent critique and history of the coronary care unit appeared in *Medical Care* (1987) 25:979. Another examination of coronary care units came from pioneer Thomas Killip, who presented his own assessment to the Conference on the Decline in Coronary Heart Disease Mortality, 1978.

10. Belated Revolution

William Roberts's paper about the role of blood clots appeared in *Circulation* (1972) 55:215. Similar findings years later were also in *Circulation* (1980) 61:219. An editorial outlining Roberts's thinking appeared in *Circulation* (1974) 59:1. Sol Sherry reviewed the history of thrombolytic therapy in the book *Thrombolytic Therapy*, edited by Anthony J. Comerota. The session with the pathologists at NIH appeared in the *American Journal of Cardiology* (1974) 34:823. Sol Sherry's comments about the results came from an interview. Three of the early streptokinase trials were in Italy, published in *Lancet* (1971) 2:891; Australia, in *Lancet* (1973) 1:57; and England, *British Medical Journal* (1976) 2:1100. The first big success with streptokinase, the European Cooperative Study Group results, was reported in *New Eng Jnl Med* (1979) 301:797. The reassessment of the role of clots urged by the Spokane group appeared in the *New Eng Jnl Med* (1980) 303:897, and an example of their surgical treatment reported in *Circulation* (1983) 68:II:12. The U.S. examination of clot breakdown by

Garrett Lee and Dean Mason was published in the *American Heart Journal* (1981) 102:783, although the first such demonstration occurred in Germany, and was reported in *Clinical Cardiology* (1981) 63:307.

The purification of TPA in usable quantities was disclosed in *Biochimica et Biophysica Acta* (1979) 580:140. Désiré Collen had produced even larger quantities from skin cancer cultures, as reported in *Journal of Biological Chemistry* (1981) 256:7035. The first cloning of TPA was retold by Genentech's Elliott B. Grossbard in Sobel, *Tissue Plasminogen Activator in Thrombolytic Therapy*, page vi. The National Institute of Health's entrance into the subject was described in the same book by the heart institute's Eugene R. Passamani, beginning at page 75.

Eugene Braunwald's declaration of thrombolytic therapy as the new frontier appeared in a two-part series in *New Eng Jnl Med*, beginning (1984) 311:710. The John Darsee episode in Braunwald's lab was reported in part in *Betrayers of the Truth* by William Broad and Nicholas Wade. More detail about the other discrepancies appeared in three articles in one edition of *Nature* (1987) Vol. 325, beginning on pages 181, 207 and 215. The two authors of a critique of the Darsee papers recount their long struggle to get a journal to publish it in *The New York Times*, April 22, 1984, page C1. Genentech's corporate fortunes were reviewed in the *Economist* April 19, 1986, page 98; in *Business Week*, April 14, 1986, page 68, and Nov. 30, 1987, page 139; the *Wall Street Journal*, June 24, 1988, page 4, October 11, 1988, page 1, and November 1, 1988, page B20. The "twice as effective" report on TPA and streptokinase appeared in *New Eng Jnl Med* (1985) 32:923. The patent claim was taken from a Genentech press release issued when the United States patent was approved. The events before the FDA advisory committee were from the transcript of the May 29, 1987, meeting. Some members of the committee later recounted their thinking in *JAMA* (1988) 2060:2250, and the *Wall Street Journal's* editorialists gave their views before the meeting, May 28, page 30, and then described their views of "The Flat Earth Committee" on July 13, 1987, page 27. The

Health Care Financing Administration response to Genentech's request for a special pass-through payment was disclosed in a Fact Sheet and Q and A released March 30, 1988. The follow-up report on the TPA/streptokinase trial at twelve months appeared in the *American Journal of Cardiology* (1988) 62:179. The most detailed comparison of the thrombolytic agents appeared in Sol Sherry's two-part series in *New Eng Jnl Med* beginning (1988) 318:1512. Genentech and Eugene Braunwald, in turn, critique Sherry's piece in letters published in *New Eng Jnl Med* (1988) 319:1543. Genentech makes some interesting points, but comes nowhere near undermining the rough equivalence of the two drugs, although with more clinical trial data it certainly would not be surprising if TPA emerged with a modest advantage.

11. LOSING THE RACE WITH DEATH

The details of Fred Forbes's cardiac arrest and resuscitation were reconstructed from interviews with Fred Forbes, Alice Forbes, Mel McClure, and Cole Kiphart, and from the incident records of the King County Emergency Medical Services.

Mickey S. Eisenberg provided two overviews of the issues and problems of sudden cardiac death outside the hospital in an article in *Scientific American* (1986) 254:37, and a book, *Sudden Cardiac Death in the Community.* Leonard A. Cobb of the University of Washington has written two excellent summaries from a medical point of view, Chapter 32 of J. Willis Hurt's textbook, *The Heart,* and the other as Chapter 9 in *The Management of the Acute Coronary Attack.* Tests on external automatic defibrillators were reported by W. Douglas Weaver in the *American Journal of Cardiology* (1986) 57:1017. Another practical overview came from John W. Bachman in *Postgraduate Medicine* (1984) 76:85. The availability of 911 service was examined by the General Accounting Office in *HRD-86-132,* "States Assume Leadership Role in Providing Emergency Services." It also examines other issues created by the end of the federal role in EMS. The original rationale for the federal role appears in the hearings for the Emergency Medical Services Act of 1973, Serial No. 93-8, Committee on Interstate and Foreign Commerce, U.S. House of Representatives. Several dozen EMS officials were interviewed for the chapter but two individuals provided the most detailed insights into the problems: Paul E. Pepe, medical director of the Houston EMS, and James O. Page, publisher of the *Journal of Emergency Medical Services,* and fire chief of Monterey Park, California.

12. No Way to Run an Airline

The error rate studies are as follows: The frequency of missed major diagnoses was described by Lee Goldman in *New Eng Jnl Med* (1983) 308:1000, and a larger autopsy survey appeared in *JAMA* (1987) 258:339. The declining autopsy rates were discussed in *JAMA* (1987) 258:364. The appropriateness of angiography was examined in *JAMA* (1987) 258:2543, and pacemakers in *New Eng Jnl Med* (1988) 318:158. Knight Steel's inquiry into iatrogenic illness appeared in *New Eng Jnl Med* (1981)304:638. The problems of legible drug orders was analyzed by Eric B. Larson in the *Western Journal of Medicine* (1983) 139:1. Handwashing was observed by Richard K. Albert in *New Eng Jnl Med* (1981) 304:1465. The accuracy of coding on Medicare hospital bills was reviewed in *New Eng Jnl Med* (1988) 318:352, and of death certificates in *American Journal of Epidemiology* (1980) 111:99.

13. A Heart Surgeon's Worst Nightmare

The account of the events at Memorial Hospital was based on interviews with the following persons: Ross Gardner, John Rubush, Mel A. Gibson, Thomas L. Poulin, Ted Beck, George V. Soaper, and Roger Birdsell. The interviews were conducted by me or Michael York in 1986 as part of a series on coronary bypass surgery written for the Knight-Ridder newspapers.

14. California Confrontation and 15. The Search for a Solution

The events at the University of California at Davis were reconstructed from the following sources:

Tape-recorded Interviews: F. William Blaisdell, Thomas Evans, Joe Tupin, Dean T. Mason, Garrett Lee, Diane Divoky, Barry Dorfman, Glen A. Lillington, Jerome Theis.

Sworn depositions: Edward J. Hurley, Todd Grehl, William Bommer, Anthony DeMaria, Reginald I. Low, Claude Smart, Kim Smith, Judy Ismach, plus Mason, Lee, and Divoky.

Documents: Approximately 1,000 pages of letters, memoranda, studies and contemporaneous notes written by Jerry P. Lewis, Ezra Amsterdam, Najam Awan, Ernest Gold, Neil Andrews, Don A. Rockwell, Joe Tupin, Tom Riemenschneider, Thomas Winston, Hibbard Williams, Glen A. Lillington, Peter M. Doyle, James A. Meyer, Elmer W. Learn, and individuals listed above. The documents were mostly legal exhibits or otherwise produced in litigation. Some were obtained by the author from the personal files of the participants.

News accounts: *Sacramento Bee, Sacramento Union, Davis Enterprise, Medical World News, San Francisco Chronicle, Time* magazine.

16. No Comparisons Needed

Henry Krakauer was interviewed for the book. Joel Brinkley revealed the existence of the list on March 3, 1986, in *The New York Times.* Philip Nathanson's comments were also from that article. Gilbert M. Gaul's story about the list appeared on page 1 of the *Philadelphia Inquirer* on March 16, 1986. JoAnn Mower's response was also from Gaul's article. Bernard Sigel's letter to the editor attacking the mortality figures appeared on page 6-G, March 23, 1986. Details of the Medical College of Pennsylvania's own internal review of bypass surgery mortality, and the concerns about competition, were revealed in a tape-recorded meeting September 12, 1986. I was present with seven senior officials of the medical college, Gilbert Gaul, and Michael York.

The Medicare mortality ranking for bypass surgery was calculated by the author from the computer tape containing the data for Krakauer's study. Washington metropolitan area mortality in open-heart surgery is disclosed in the 1986 Annual Report: "Specialized Cardiac Care Services in the Washington Metropolitan Area." The tables cover mortality experience since 1980.

APPENDIX:
BRAND AND GENERIC
DRUG NAMES

Brand Name	Generic Name
Activase	recombinant TPA or alteplase, recombinant
Aribrate	clofibrate
Atromid-S	clofibrate
Choloxin	dextrothyroxine
Colestid	colestipol hydrochloride
Lopid	gemfibrozil
Lorelco	probucol
MER /29	triparanol
Mevacor	lovastatin
Nicolar	niacin
Nicotinex	niacin compound
Questran	cholestyramine resin
Streptase	streptokinase
Valium	diazepam

BIBLIOGRAPHY

Ackerknecht, Erwin A. *A Short History of Medicine.* Baltimore: Johns Hopkins University Press, 1982.

American Hospital Association. *American Hospital Association Guide to the Health Care Field.* Chicago: American Hospital Association, 1986.

Anderson, Jeffrey L. *Acute Myocardial Infarction, New Management Strategies.* Rockville, Maryland: Aspen Publications, 1987.

Baldry, P.E. *The Battle Against Heart Disease.* Boston: Cambridge University Press, 1971.

Bourke, Jeoffrey J., Leslie E. Daly and James McGilvray. *Interpretation and Uses of Medical Statistics.* Oxford, England: Blackwell Scientific Publications, 1985.

Broad, William and Nicholas Wade. *Betrayers of the Truth.* New York: Simon and Schuster, Inc., 1982.

Bunker, J.P., Benjamin A. Barnes and Frederick Mosteller. *Costs, Risks and Benefits of Surgery.* New York: Oxford University Press, 1977.

Callahan, Daniel. *Setting Limits: Medical Goals in an Aging Society.* New York: Simon & Schuster, 1987.

Carlson, Rick J. *The End of Medicine.* New York: Wiley & Sons, 1975.

Chung, Edward K. *Cardiac Emergency Care.* Philadelphia: Lee & Febiger, 1980.

Comerota, Anthony J., ed. *Thrombolytic Therapy.* Orlando, FL: Grune & Stratton, Inc., 1988.

Cooper, Kenneth H. *Controlling Cholesterol.* New York: Bantam Books, 1988.

Dawber, Thomas Royle. *The Framingham Study.* Cambridge, MA: Harvard University Press, 1980.

Doby, T., M.D. *Discoverers of Blood Circulation.* New York: Abelard-Schuman Limited, 1963.

Dubos, Rene. *Mirage of Health.* New York: Harper & Row, 1959. Perennial Library edition.

Duncan, R. and M. Weston-Smith, editors. *The Encyclopaedia of Medical Ignorance.* London: Pergamon Press, 1984.

Dutton, Dianna B. *Worse than the Disease: Pitfalls of Medical Progress.* New York: Cambridge University Press, 1988.

Eger, Joel H., James T. Niemann, Keith G. Bowman, and J. Michael Criley. *Cardiology for the House Officer.* Baltimore: Williams & Wilkins, 1982.

Eisenberg, Mickey S., Lawrence Bergner and Alfred P. Hallstrom. *Sudden Cardiac Death in the Community.* New York: Praeger Publishers, 1984.

Executive Office of the President. *Budget of the United States Government, Fiscal Year 1988.* Washington, D.C.: U.S. Government Printing Office, 1987.

Fine, Ralph Adam. *The Great Drug Deception.* New York: Stein and Day, 1972.

Fowler, Noble O. *Cardiac Diagnosis and Treatment.* Philadelphia: Harper & Row, 1980.

Fox, John P., Carrie E. Hall and Lila R. Elveback. *Epidemiology, Man and Disease.* New York: Macmillan Co., 1970.

Fuchs, Victor R. *Who Shall Live?* New York: Basic Books, 1974.

General Accounting Office. *States Assume Leadership Role in Providing Emergency Services.* Washington, D.C.: General Accounting Office, Pub. HRD-86-132, 1986.

Gutkind, Lee. *Many Sleepless Nights.* New York: W.W. Norton, 1988.

Guyton, Arthur C. *Textbook of Medical Physiology.* Philadelphia: W.B. Saunders Company, 1986.

Hall, Stephen S. *Invisible Frontiers.* New York: Atlantic Monthly Press, 1987.

Health Care Financing Administration. *A Model for Prediction of Statistical Outliers.* Baltimore: Health Care Financing Administration, 1986.

Hersey, Nathan. *Hospital-Physician Relationships.* Rockville, Md: Aspen Systems Corporation, 1982.

Hiatt, Howard H. *America's Health in the Balance.* New York: Harper & Row, 1987.

Hurst, J. Willis, editor-in-chief. *The Heart.* New York: McGraw-Hill, 1986.

Illich, Ivan. *Medical Nemesis.* New York: Pantheon Books, 1975.

Inlander, Charles B., Lowell S. Levin and Ed Weiner. *Medicine on Trial.* New York: Prentice Hall Press, 1988.

Jang, G. David. *Angioplasty.* New York: McGraw-Hill Book Company, 1986.

Joint Commission of Accredition of Healthcare Organizations. *Accreditation Manual for Hospitals.* Chicago: Joint Commission on Accreditation of Healthcare Organizations, 1987.

Kent, George C. *Comparative Anatomy of the Vertebrates.* St. Louis: C.V. Mosby Company, 1983.

King, Spencer B., III and John S. Douglas, Jr. *Coronary Arteriography and Angioplasty.* New York: McGraw-Hill Book Company, 1985.

Kowalski, Robert A. *The 8-Week Cholestrol Cure.* New York: Harper & Row, 1987.

Metropolitan Washington Area Council of Health Planning Agencies. *Specialized Cardiac Care Services in the Metropolitan Washington Area, 1986 Annual Report.* Washington, D.C.: Metropolitan Washington Area Council of Health Planning Agencies, 1988.

National Center for Health Statistics. *Detailed Diagnoses and Surgical Procedures for Patients Discharged from Short Stay Hospitals: 1987.* Washington, D.C.: National Center for Health Statistics, 1988.

National Institutes of Health. *Hypertension Prevalence and the Status of Awareness, Treatment and Control in the United States, Final Report of the Subcommittee on Definition and Prevalence of the Joint National Committee on Detection, Evaluation and Treatment of High Blood Pressure.* Bethesda, MD: National Institutes of Health, 1984.

Payer, Lynn. *Medicine & Culture.* New York: Henry Holt & Company, New York, 1988.

Pines, Maya. *Inside the Cell.* DHEW Pub. No. (NIH) 79-1051, 1979.

Riegelman, Richard K., M.D. *Studying a Study, Testing a Test.* Boston: Little, Brown and Company, 1981.

Rothman, Kenneth J. *Modern Epidemiology.* Boston: Little, Brown and Company, 1986.

Rowlands, Derek J. *Recent Advances in Cardiology-10.* Edinburgh: Churchill-Livingston, 1987.

Sagan, Leonard A. *The Health of Nations.* New York: Basic Books, 1987.

Siegel, Bernie S. *Love, Medicine & Miracles.* New York: Harper & Row, 1986.

Sobel, Burton E., Désiré Collen and Elliot B. Grossbard. *Tissue Plasminogen Activator in Thrombolytic Therapy.* New York: Marcel Dekker, Inc., 1987.

Starr, Paul. *The Social Transformation of Medicine.* New York: Basic Books, 1984.

Thomas, Lewis. *The Youngest Science.* New York: The Viking Press, 1983.

Thomas, Lewis. *The Lives of a Cell.* New York: The Viking Press, 1974.

U.S. Department of Health, Education and Welfare. *Proceedings of the Conference on the Decline in Coronary Heart Disease Mortality.* Washington, D.C.: NIH Pub. No. 79-1610, May, 1979.

U.S. Department of Health, Education and Welfare. *The Framingham Study: An Epidemiological Investigation of Cardiovascular Disease.* DHEW Pub. No. (NIH) 74-618,74-478,74-599,76-1083.

U.S. Department of Health, Education and Welfare. *Arteriosclerosis: A Report by the National Heart Lung and Blood Institute Task Force on Arteriosclerosis.* DHEW Pub. No. (NIH) 72-137, June 1971.

Wake, Marvalee H., ed. *Hyman's Comparative Vertebrate Anatomy.* Chicago: University of Chicago Press, third edition, 1979.

Walmsley, Robert and Hamish Watson. *Clinical Anatomy of the Heart.* Edinburgh: Churchill-Livingston, 1978.

Wertenbaker, Lael. *To Mend the Heart.* New York: Viking, 1980.

White, Paul Dudley. *My Life in Medicine.* Boston: Gambit Inc., 1971.

Woolf, Neville. *Pathology of Atherosclerosis.* London: Butterworth Scientific, 1982.

Woolson, Robert W. *Statistical Methods for the Analysis of Biomedical Data.* New York: John Wiley & Sons, 1987.

INDEX

About the Author

THOMAS J. MOORE has spent twenty years investigating and writing about public problems. He has explored issues ranging from the breakdown in truck safety to why so many recent college graduates can't get good jobs. Moore has probed government corruption as a prize-winning reporter for the *Chicago Sun-Times*, and investigated the CIA for a U.S. Senate committee. As a national correspondent in the Washington Bureau of Knight-Ridder newspapers he documented why unnecessary deaths occur in coronary bypass surgery. The series won reporting awards from National Press Club, the White House Correspondents Association, and the National Headliners' Club. He is currently a visiting fellow at the Graduate Institute for Policy Education and Research, George Washington University, and lives in Washington, D.C.